Francisco Pantoja Braga
Francisco P. Braga Filho
Rebeca P. Braga

Impression Taking in Implant Prosthodontics

Francisco Pantoja Braga
Francisco P. Braga Filho
Rebeca P. Braga

Impression Taking in Implant Prosthodontics

Evaluation of the Accuracy of 4 Techniques

ScienciaScripts

This book is a translation from the original published under ISBN 978-613-9-62605-2.

Publisher:
Sciencia Scripts
is a trademark of
Dodo Books Indian Ocean Ltd. and OmniScriptum S.R.L publishing group

120 High Road, East Finchley, London, N2 9ED, United Kingdom
Str. Armeneasca 28/1, office 1, Chisinau MD-2012, Republic of Moldova, Europe
Printed at: see last page
ISBN: 978-620-7-74600-2

Summary

I dedicate this work to

To my children, **Francisco Filho** and **Rebeca**,
for being the main reason for my
moments of inspiration and happiness.

Special thanks

To **Prof. Dr. Guilherme Elias Pessanha Henriques,** by whom I had the honor of being supervised. My sincere thanks for all the trust you have placed in me, for your teachings, for your patience, tolerance and understanding during this period. Thank you very much.

To **Vanessa Silva Tramontino**, for her indispensable assistance in understanding and carrying out the extensometry and microscopy. Thank you for your attention and friendship.

To FAPEAM - **Fundaçâo de Amparo à Pesquisa do Estado do Amazonas,** for the financial support provided during my studies in Piracicaba.

My thanks

To the State University of Campinas (UNICAMP), in the person of its Magnificent Rector **José Tadeu Jorge**.

To the Piracicaba School of Dentistry of the State University of Campinas (FOP-UNICAMP), in the person of its Director **Prof. Dr. Francisco Haiter Neto** and Associate Director *Prof. Dr. Marcelo de Castro Meneghim.*

To **Prof. Dr. Jacks Jorge Jûnior**, Coordinator of the Postgraduate Courses at FOP-UNICAMP and **Prof. Dr. Renata Cunha Matheus Rodrigues Garcia**, Coordinator of the Postgraduate Course in Clinical Dentistry at FOP-UNICAMP.

To the University of the State of Amazonas (UEA), in the person of its Magnificent Rector *Marilene Corrêa da Silva Freitas*.

To the coordinators of the Dentistry Course at UEA, **Prof. Dr. Tânia Miranda Chicre Alcantara and Prof. Dr. Benedito Taveira dos Santos,** for their support at all times when I needed to be absent from my teaching activities.

To the members of the Qualifying Board, *Prof. Dr. Marcelo Ferraz Mesquita, Prof. Dr. Simonides Consani, Prof. Dr. Rafael Leonardo Xediek Consani,* for their considerations and suggestions for improving this work.

To all the professors of the Minter/Dinter course in Clinical Dentistry at FOP-UNICAMP, who contributed greatly to my learning during this stage of my life.

To my friends at Repùblica da Primavera, *Ligia Vasconcelos, Alexandra Pieri, Jonas Alves, Joelson Brum, Naelca Sarmento and Ana Lucia Diefenbach*, for their pleasant interaction and companionship.

To *Sandra Premoli*, for her love, affection, understanding, support and encouragement.

To all the Minter/Dinter colleagues, for the interaction and exchange of experiences during the seminars in Manaus.

To my colleagues at FOP, *Leonardo Luthi, Aloisio Spazzin, Juliana Nunez* and *Gessica Takahashi,* for the pleasant interaction during this period.

To the secretary of the Department of Prosthodontics and Periodontics, *Eliete Ap. F. L. Marim,* and to the interns, *Mônica L. B. Penzani and Suelen Sarto,* for their sympathy, attention and help during my postgraduate studies.

To all those who indirectly contributed to this work.

Summary

This *in vitro* study aimed to evaluate the accuracy of four molding techniques for osseointegrated implants. A superstructure simulating a prosthesis was constructed from a metal matrix containing three implants. The four techniques studied were separated as follows: Group A - 10 impressions with conical transfers (without bonding) in closed individual trays; Group B - 10 impressions with isolated square transfers in open trays; Group C - 10 impressions with square transfers bonded with self-curing resin in open individual trays; Group D - 10 impressions with square transfers bonded with self-curing Bis-acrylic composite resin in open individual trays. The impression material for all groups was Honigum Mono (DMG) silicone and the plaster used to make the models was Resin Rock (Whip Mix-USA). Marginal misalignments were assessed between the metal superstructure screwed to the working models obtained from the impressions using an optical microscope (120X magnification), as well as the stresses induced in the superstructure, assessed by extensometry. The Kruskal-Wallis non-parametric test was used to compare the groups, with a significance level of 5%, to check for significant differences between the groups with regard to the two variables studied. Multiple non-parametric comparisons were used to indicate which group or groups led to statistical significance. The Kruskal-Wallis test showed a p-value of 0.0043 for the **tension variable** and 0.6073 for the **misfit** variable. With 5% being the level set, it was possible to observe that only for the **tension variable did** the groups show a significant difference between them. Pearson's correlation coefficient was calculated for the **tension** and **maladjustment** variables, indicating a positive correlation between the variables. This correlation was highly significant (p=0.0074). The other values found were not statistically significant. It was concluded that the most accurate of the four techniques studied was the one that used square transfers splinted with pre-made resin rods and that there was a direct correlation between marginal misfit and stresses generated in the superstructure.

Keywords: Dental impression technique; dental implant; dental models.

1. Introduction

New types of prostheses have emerged since osseointegration was proven in the works of Branemark *et al.,* 1977; Albrektsson et *al.,* 1981; Adell *et al.,* 1981, demonstrating scientifically and irrefutably that the use of titanium screws with endosseous fixation could be used reliably as a support for various types of rehabilitative prosthetic treatment.

With the new restorative prosthetic modalities, the passivity or passive adaptation of prosthetic structures has become a common concern in prosthetic rehabilitation. Passive adaptation, or passivity, of an implant-retained prosthesis is assumed to be the situation in which this prosthesis adapts with the least possible marginal misfit and in a passive manner to the retaining component, without creating stresses on the implant itself or the surrounding bone tissue (Millington and Leung, 1995).

Due to the biological and biomechanical characteristics of osseointegration, it is thought that any stress generated on an osseointegrated fixture will be directly transferred to the supporting bone tissues due to the lack of relative mobility between the system's structures (Skalak, 1983). A poorly adapted prosthesis rigidly connected to multiple implants can exert extremely high levels of stress on the fixtures and, consequently, on the tissues that support them (Jemt and Lekholm, 1998).

It has been reported that biological and mechanical problems may be related to the lack of passive adaptation of the prosthetic structure on the abutments or implants (Zarb and Schmitt, 1991; Naert *et al.,* 1992; Adell et al., 1981; Bauman et *al.,* 1992).

Authors such as Zarb and Schmitt, 1991; Naert *et al.,* 1992, have observed a positive correlation between the incidence of mechanical problems and the presence of marginal misalignments in prostheses on implants. The most commonly reported mechanical complications are loosening or fracture of the screws holding the prostheses to the connecting abutments, fracture of the abutments themselves, the prosthetic structure or even the fixings. It is also thought that this type of failure can prematurely reveal a lack of passive seating, overloading the entire system. Biological complications such as adverse reaction of the surrounding tissues, pain, pressure sensation, peri-implant bone resorption and even complete failure of osseointegration (Adell *et al.,* 1981; Bauman *et al.,* 1992) are also related to a lack of passive adaptation.

A structure with a passive fit should theoretically induce zero stress in the implant components and the surrounding bone in the absence of an applied external load. However, an absolutely passive structure has not been achieved in the last three decades

(Sahin and Çehreli, 2001

The main purpose of a bone-integrated implant impression, apart from recording and transferring, is to reproduce the relationship between the implants as accurately as possible. They also serve the secondary but important purpose of recording soft tissue morphology (Gregory-Head and Labarre, 1999; Wee, 2000 and Goiato *et al.*, 2002). In the Branemark system, there are conical and square transfers that lend themselves to this purpose and which adapt to intermediates and their replicas. However, there are varying techniques for using them, resulting in research that seeks to identify the superiority of one technique over another (Goiato *et al.*, 1998).

Humphries *et al.* in 1990 concluded that the technique with conical transfers is better than the technique with square transfers bonded or not with acrylic resin. In contrast, Carr, 1991; Fenton *et al., 1991*; Rodney *et al.,* 1991 and Phillips *et al.*, 1994 concluded that the technique with square transfers is better than that with conical transfers. However, Carr, 1992; Goiato et *al.*, 1998; Herbst et *al.,* 2000; Pinto et *al.,* 2001; Goiato *et al.,* 2002 and Naconecy et *al.,* 2004 concluded that they are the same.

Fenton *et al.*, 1991; Assif *et al.*, 1996; Vigolo et al., 2003; Assunçâo et *al.,* 2004; Naconecy *et al.,* 2004 and Cabral, 2005, Rodrigues,2006, De'Acqua *et al.,* 2008, advocate bonding the square transfers with acrylic resin to make the transfer impressions, thus obtaining the best results. However, research by Humphries *et al.*, 1990; Spector et *al.,* 1990; Hsu et *al.,* 1993; Inturregui et *al.,* 1993; Phillips *et al.,* 1994; Burawi et *al.,* 1997; Goiato *et al.,* 1998; Goiato *et al.,* 2002; Herbst*et al.,* 2000 and Pinto et *al.*, 2001 have shown that the joining of the transferors is unnecessary.

There is no consensus on the most precise implant transfer molding technique.

A new material has recently emerged, suitable for making crowns, inlays, onlays and long-term temporary fixed prostheses. It is a self-curing composite based on multifunctional methacrylates, presented in the form of a cartridge with self-mixing tips to be used in an appropriate gun, which characterizes its practicality of use. Due to its characteristics, the possibility of using it in the joining of transfers was suggested, comparing this technique with other existing ones.

Several methods can be used to compare impression techniques for implant-supported prostheses, as reported in the literature: Using resin rods to bond the transfers (Humphries *et al.,* 1990; Carr and Sokol, 19991; Fenton *et al.*, 1991; Rodney et *al.,* 1991; Assif et *al.*,1992; Carr, 1992; Phillips et al., 1994; Pinto et *al.,* 2001; Goiato *et al.,* 2002; Assunçâo, et *al.,* 2004; Rodrigues, 2006; Del'Acqua, *et al.,* 2008); using acrylic resin on dental floss to bond the transfers (Spector *et al.,* 1990; Hsu et *al., 1993;* Inturregui et *al.,* 1993; Assif *et al.,* 1996; Burawi et al., 1997; Gennari Filho *et al.,* 2009); using light-curing composite resin (Ivanhoe, *et al.,* 2006) using plaster for molding (Inturregui et *al.,* 1993; Assif, *et al.,* 1999; Wise, 1991); using self-curing acrylic resin and self-curing composite resin (Augustin *et al.,* 2009); isolated cones and squares (Carr and Sokol, 1991; Carr, 1991; Carr, 1992; Rodney *et al.,* 1991).

However, there has been no research evaluating or correlating marginal misalignments and stresses induced in the superstructure at the same time.

The aim of this research was to study four transfer molding techniques *in vitro* to see which was the most accurate, after evaluating marginal misalignments under microscopy and stresses induced by extensometry on a metal superstructure.

The following hypotheses were evaluated in this study:

1)   That a transfer molding technique using a new material will be superior to existing ones;

2)   That there is a direct correlation between the variables misalignment and tension.

2. Literature review

Humphries *et al.* (1990) carried out a comparative study of three impression techniques with BRANEMARK implants, by checking the accuracy of the models obtained. They used an aluminum metal matrix simulating the dimensions of a mandible with four abutment analogs. Four reference points were milled into the metal matrix. Individual molds made of self-curing and lightened resin were used to make the impressions, with the two-step technique, using a silicone-based material by addition (President, Coltene). The three transfer techniques were: 1- conical transfers; 2- square transfers; 3- square transfers bonded with Duralay resin (30 min before the impression was taken). The impression was taken with the model at a temperature of 37°C, simulating a clinical situation. The molds were removed after eight minutes of polymerization in a water bath at this temperature. Four molds were taken for each technique. The implant analogs were adapted to the transfers and the mold filled with Vel-Mix plaster. Four special pins were adapted to the models obtained for measurement using a computerized graphic measuring system, with an accuracy of ± 3μm, in the spatial coordinates (x, y, z). The average values and standard deviations of each of the reference points on the twelve models were compared with the values for each point on the metal model. The authors concluded that when compared to the original model, the reference points showed values with no statistically significant difference or values consistent with the dimensional changes of the materials used. Using conical transfers, 92% of the values were not significantly different from those of the metal model. With unsplinted and splinted square transfers respectively, 50% and 42% of the values were not significantly different from those of the metal model. Of the three techniques, that of the conical transfers had a numerical difference of less than 50 μm 100% of the time. The unsplinted and splinted square transfers had a numerical difference of less than 50 μm 59% and 58% of the time, respectively. The indirect technique with conical transfers reproduced the experimental points better than the other techniques.

Mojon *et al.* (1990) verified the inadequate dimensional stability caused by polymerization contraction in relation to the various applications of acrylic resins. The aim of the study was to evaluate and compare dimensional changes of two self-curing acrylic resins marketed as standard and index materials and to analyze the influence of the powder-to-liquid ratio. Initial volumetric changes (2 min to 17 min after mixing) were measured with a dilatometer and later linear changes (from 17 min to 24 hours or more) were recorded with an inductive transducer. The time of the two experiments was determined based on preliminary tests. After 24 hours the volumetric contraction was 7.9% for Duralay resin and 6.5% for Palavit G resin; 80% of the changes appeared before 17 minutes at room temperature; 95% before 3 hours for Duralay resin and 2 hours for Palavit G resin. No statistical difference was found up to 17 min between the two materials. Up to 24 hours, the linear shrinkage of Palavit G resin was significantly lower than that of Duralay resin for mixtures of similar consistencies (Linear shrinkage as a function of the consistency of thick, standard and fluid resin for Palavit G: 0.29%, 0.34% and 0.41% and for Duralay: 0.37%, 0.47% and 0.49% respectively). Shrinkage was significantly increased when the proportion of powder in the mixture was decreased. The results suggest that these resins should be used with some method to compensate for shrinkage when used as an index material. It is advisable to re-bond the indexes when almost all polymerization contraction has occurred. Using as thick a mixture as possible will also minimize the worst effects of polymerization. However, the dimensional change could provide significant advantages for intracoronal moldings.

Spector *et al.* (1990) evaluated three transfer molding techniques for osseointegrated implants with multiple measurements. A model simulating a mandible with six implants was used, reproduced using three transfer techniques. Technique I - individual acrylic resin tray with upper opening, square transfers joined with acrylic resin (Duralay) and dental floss and molded with polysulfide. Technique II - stock trays, cylindrical transfers and molding with polyvinylsiloxane. Technique III - stock trays, cylindrical transfers and molding with condensation silicon. All the components used were from Nobelpharma. Five molds and five models were made with each technique (cast in improved stone plaster). Six cylindrical transfers were machined on their upper surface to allow measurements to be made on the X-Y axis (horizontal plane) and Z axis (vertical axis). The authors concluded that the magnitude of the distortions was similar in the three techniques evaluated.

Jemt (1991) followed up 391 fixed maxillary and mandibular total prostheses for one year, supported by 2199 implants, and obtained success rates of 99.5% and 98.1% for the prostheses and implants, respectively. Although complications were few, they were more frequent in the maxilla. Among the complications encountered, the following stood out: diction problems (31.2%), lip and jugal mucosa bite (6.6%), irritation caused by the cantilever (3.1%), gingival problems (fistula, hyperplasia, inflammation - 1.7%), fracture of the metal structure (0.8%). None of the components fractured. With regard to loosening of the gold screws, the author reported that 271 prostheses (69.3%) had stable screws in the first control (after 2 weeks), and almost all the screws retightened in this first control were stable in the next control (after 3 months). Only 7 prostheses needed more than one retightening for the screws to stabilize. A protocol was suggested for analyzing the adaptation of the prosthesis: considering a fixed prosthesis supported by five implants, numbered 1 to 5 from left to right, the prosthesis should be positioned and screw 1 tightened completely. This checks the fit of the other end component. The procedure should be repeated with the other distal screw (screw 5). Once the fit has been checked, all the screws are tightened one at a time, starting with screw 2, then screw 4, then the intermediate screw and eventually the two distal screws. Each screw should be tightened to its first resistance, noting the position of the wrench and a maximum of half a turn (180°) should be made on the wrench for the final tightening (10 to 15 Ncm). Another way of assessing adaptation was by the number of turns made during the tightening of the gold screw. When more than half a turn was needed to completely tighten the screw, the structure was considered to be poorly adapted and was sectioned and welded.

Carr & Sokol (1991) reported that working models should accurately represent the intra-oral relationship of the implants to enable the fabrication of passive fit prostheses. In this study, they compared the accuracy of the models (obtained from a partially edentulous model with two Nobelpharma implants positioned parallel and placed in the right posterior region) using two implant transfer molding techniques - direct (square transfers) and indirect (conical transfers). A metal frame was used to obtain measurements (mm) by tightening the anterior implant with a constant torque (14 in. oz.). Four 1.57 mm stainless steel balls were placed in the framework: two buccally and two lingually. The four spheres corresponding to the master model were transferred by the molds (made with a polyether: Caulk Polygel) to the experimental models (Whip Mix - Prima Rock) allowing four measurements to be made between pairs of spheres. Nine models were produced for each technique and the data was obtained using a microscope (precision 0.003 mm). The absolute average observed minus the predicted values was 0.070 mm for the indirect technique and 0.020 mm for the direct technique. Under the conditions of this study, there is no convincing evidence that one technique is more accurate than the other.

In 1991, Carr reported that the production of an accurate metal framework that satisfies the implant dentistry objective of passive fit requires an understanding of potential processing errors. The accuracy of working models fabricated by molding using two different Nobelpharma transfers was investigated. A plaster model representing a mandible with five implant abutments located in the anterior region was used to produce seven models for both the indirect and direct transfer techniques. The divergence angles between abutments were all less than 15°. An individual tray made of acrylic resin (Formatray, Kerr) with polyether (Polygel, LD Caulk/Dentsply) was used to make the impressions. The variability of the repeated screw fixations for the indirect and direct transfer components was ≤ 20 µm. The comparison was made using a metal structure adapted for the master model. Differences in the distances measured between each group and the master model were analyzed. For the model used, the direct technique produced more accurate working models. The inaccuracy seen with the indirect transfer method seemed to be related to the non-parallelism between the abutments (< 15 degrees) and the apparent deformation of the impression material.

Fenton *et al.* (1991) carried out a study comparing the accuracy of implant models produced using four different transfer molding techniques. A metal framework for a standard mandibular implant prosthesis was made and then a metal model of a mandibular arch with five implants (Nobelpharma) was made to fit it. Fifteen models were obtained for each of the four transfer molding techniques. The fit of the prefabricated metal framework for each model was assessed manually. Then, the difference between passive seating and adaptation by screw tightening was measured under a microscope at 30x magnification. The results for the transfer impression techniques were: a - square transfers bonded with acrylic resin and molded with alginate (0 with worst fit / gap 4.17 µm); b - square transfers bonded with acrylic resin and molded with polyether (0 with worst fit / gap 4.17 µm); c - square transfers without bonding and molding with polyether (4 with worst fit / gap 11 µm); d - conical transfers and molding with silicone by addition (8 with worst fit / gap 21.6 µm). Manual assessment of passive fit correlated with gap measurements. When acrylic resin was used to bond the square transfers, all the models were acceptable and more accurate than the best result obtained with the other techniques, regardless of the impression material used.

Ivanhoe *et al.* (1991) described a transfer molding technique for implants with joined square transfers. They used a patient with five implants fixed in the mandible, where a preliminary impression was taken with cylindrical transfers and irreversible hydrocolloid. Once the model was obtained, the cylindrical transfers were replaced by square transfers. A rigid connection was made between them with light-curing resin, leaving 1 mm of space between each transfer. After this procedure, the resin transfers were removed from the model and adapted to the intraoral implants, receiving a torque of 10 Ncm and then bonded with light-curing resin of gel consistency, before the impression was taken. The authors concluded that this technique reduced clinical time by eliminating the need for floss and Duralay, minimized changes during polymerization by reducing the amount of resin and reduced discomfort for the patient.

Rodney *et al.* (1991) reported that the manufacturing process of implant prostheses involves the critical transfer of intraoral records to laboratory models. Any dimensional alteration in this process can lead to poor final results or complete failure of the prosthesis. They evaluated the dimensional accuracy between two transfer molding systems for implants (Branemark System, Nobelpharma): square transfers (direct) and conical transfers (indirect). A standard model was fabricated with two replica abutments fixed with epoxy resin. Individual molds were used to make the impressions with polyether (Impregum). Twelve models were obtained for both transfer molding systems and the measurements were taken directly on the models using a measuring microscope (Nikon). The results showed that the average dimension between the replicas of the standard model abutments was 0.6758 inches with a possible measurement error of 0.0002 inches. The conical transfers had an average value of 0.6808 inches with a standard deviation of 0.0023 inches and the square transfers had an average value of 0.6778 inches with a standard deviation of 0.0017 inches. The authors concluded that transfer molding with the square transfer (direct) was dimensionally more accurate than with the conical transfer (indirect).

Assif *et al.* (1992) compared the dimensional accuracy of four different transfer molding procedures for osseointegrated implants. A special stone plaster mandibular model with five implant analogues was constructed for this study. A metal structure (representative of a mandibular implant prosthesis) was waxed up and cast. This structure was the standard for all measurements during the evaluation of the accuracy of the models obtained by the different impression procedures. Analogs were screwed to the metal structure and then included inside the aluminum block with epoxy resin. This formed a metal model that already had a metal framework passively fitted to it. Four transfer molding techniques were used: 1- metal stock tray with top opening and sealed with wax base plate, square transfers bonded with Duralay resin 24 hours before, but with a 1 mm gap between each transfer, which were bonded 15 min before the alginate impression was taken; 2- individual acrylic resin tray, square transfers joined with Duralay resin (in the same way as in technique 1) and molded with polyether; 3- individual acrylic resin tray, square transfers without joining and molded with polyether; 4- perforated metal stock tray, conical transfers, molding with polyvinylsiloxane (double mixing technique). Fifteen models were obtained for each technique. The criterion used to check the accuracy of the moldings was the fit of the anatolgals in each model to the metal structure. This was judged manually as well as visually using a microscope. The metal framework was seated on each model and digital pressure was applied alternately to the regions corresponding to the top of each of the five implants. Two examiners made their observations independently and then compared the results. Visual analysis was carried out using a microscope with 30x magnification. A guide screw was tightened on the central implant to keep the structure in a constant position while measurements were taken on the end cylinders (the discrepancy that existed due to the impression procedures was determined by the difference in distance when the cylinder was unscrewed from when it was tightened with the screw). Two measurements were taken for each of the two end abutments. When the transfers were bonded with acrylic resin (techniques 1 and 2), all thirty models were judged to be passively adapted to the structure and were assumed to be clinically acceptable (average misadaptation of 4.17 μm). In technique 3, eleven of the fifteen models were judged to be passively and clinically acceptable (the average maladaptation in the fifteen models was 11 μm). When conical transfers were used (technique 4), only seven of the fifteen models were judged to be clinically acceptable (the average maladjustment in the fifteen models was 21.6 μm). There was a clear correlation between the clinical assessment of passive fit and the discrepancy measured under the microscope. The authors concluded that when acrylic resin was used to bond the transfers (techniques 1 and 2), all the models were acceptable and more accurate than the best of the other two techniques. When this was not done, the square transfers gave good results. Most of the models produced with technique 4 (conical transfers) were considered unacceptable.

Carr (1992) reported that when working with implants, it is necessary to understand the importance of the accuracy and precision of all the fabrication and joining phases in order to achieve a suprastructure that passively fits the implants. The author evaluated the accuracy of working models produced from impressions using two different transfers (conical and square). To do this, a master mandibular model was built, partially edentulous, with two implants positioned in the left posterior region, 11 mm apart from center to center, the anterior one parallel to the adjacent 1st premolar and the posterior one with a 15 degree lingual inclination. A relief of 2 mm was made around the teeth and implant transfers to make the individual impression trays. The impression material used for both techniques was polyether (Polygel - Caulk/Dentsply). Ten models were made for each technique. The transfer was considered effective in the production of models if the distance between specific points on the models agreed with the corresponding distance on the master model. The absolute value of the difference in distances between experimental and master models was compared for the two techniques. No statistically significant differences were noted. Both techniques provide comparable results with an average discrepancy value of 36 µm and 35 µm for direct and indirect transfer, respectively. This suggests that there is no clear advantage in using the direct method in clinical situations similar to those studied.

Hsu *et al.* (1993) evaluated and compared the accuracy with which the position of the abutments was reproduced in four different implant transfer techniques using two model-making systems. An experimental stainless steel analog with two implants and anterior and two posterior abutments was fabricated. Individual acrylic resin trays (Formatray) were made with two wax blades. All the techniques used square transfers, as follows: technique I - square transfers only; II - bonded with Duralay and dental floss; III - 0.03" diameter orthodontic stainless steel wire bonded with Duralay; IV - prefabricated Duralay resin blocks around the transfers that were effectively splinted with a small amount of resin. All resin splinting was done 20 minutes before impression taking. Impregum adhesive was applied to the individual trays 15 min before the final impression. Fourteen impressions were taken according to each Impregum transfer technique, for a total of fifty-six impressions. To simulate the intraoral condition, the experimental analog was kept in a humidified oven at 37° C for 10 min before taking the impression. The impression material was allowed to polymerize for 15 min in an oven at 32° C before separation. The guide pins were unscrewed and the impressions were separated from the experimental analog. Replicas of the brass abutments were attached to the transfers and held in place by the guide pins. The fourteen impressions from each technique were divided into two equal groups, seven each, as follows: Group 1 - solid model (Fujirock) vacuum-blasted for 40 seconds, waiting for a 60-minute setting period and kept at room temperature for at least 24 hours before measurements were taken; Group 2- Zeiser system (die-cast model). The measurements were taken with a profile projector (Nikon, model H-14B, Tokyo, Japan). Each model was removed from the profile projector and replaced between readings (three for each model). Two horizontal measurements were taken (between the posterior AD and anterior BC abutments) and four vertical measurements were taken at the height of each abutment (A,B,C,D). There was no statistically significant interaction between the implant transfer techniques and the master model systems used. Average AD= 40.67 to 58.49 µm and BC= 50.73 to 66.86 µm. Significant differences were only observed between the vertical changes of pillars B and D subjected to transfer techniques II and IV. Between the solid and die-cast model systems (Zeiser) there was some statistically significant difference: solid AD= 61.28 µm and die-cast AD= 39.42 µm; solid C= 38.49 µm and die-cast C= 22.66 µm; solid D= 38.55 µm and die-cast D= 21.41 µm. For all practical purposes, it seems that the non-splinted technique using a suitable impression material can reduce some of the complexity of the transfer procedures and save clinical time. The Zeiser system tends to minimize distortions of abutment positions attributable to plaster expansion. The authors conclude that: 1- The volume of Duralay acrylic resin used to bond the transfers is an insignificant factor in the accuracy of the transfer impressions. 2- There is no significant difference in the accuracy of the transfer impressions between the splinted and unsplinted techniques. 3- With the Zeiser system it was possible to achieve a reduction in errors between abutments in the posterior region of master models when compared to a solid model system.

Skalak (1993) analyzed the macroscopic stress distribution and load transfer mechanisms where the intimate juxtaposition of bone on titanium implants is provided at the microscopic level. It also presented some qualitative guidelines regarding implant positioning and the mode of action that can be expected from fixed partial dentures on osseointegrated implants. The conclusions were as follows: 1- The intimate juxtaposition of bone to the titanium implant is the essential characteristic that allows stress to be transmitted from the implant to the bone without any appreciable relative movement or abrasion. The absence of any fibrotic interlayer allows the stress to be transmitted without any progressive change in the union or contact between bone and implant; 2- The use of a threaded screw provides a form of engagement with the bone on a macroscopic scale that allows the full development of the bone's resistance to shear or compression. A smooth, cylindrical implant may require an adhesive bond for satisfactory performance, but a screw-shaped one can work whether or not a true adhesive bond is developed, as long as the juxtaposition of bone and implant is intimate; 3- The distribution of a vertical or lateral load applied to a fixed partial denture depends on the number, arrangement and hardness of the abutments used, as well as the shape and hardness of the fixed partial denture itself.

In general, a rigid fixed partial denture will distribute loads to several implants more effectively. A flexible prosthesis may be suitable if the resistance developed by each implant can transmit the total load that is applied. Fixed partial dentures with cantilevers increase the load on the first screw closest to the cantilever. Moderate projections (of the cantilever) can be tolerated if the implants are strong enough; 4- A tight connection between the fixed partial denture and the implants provides a single structure that can act in combination with the bone to provide greater strength than the implants or the mandibular bone alone; 5- Osseointegrated implants provide direct contact with the bone and will thus transmit any stress waves or shocks applied to the implants. It is therefore advisable to use a damping material such as acrylic resin in the artificial teeth used in fixed partial dentures. This arrangement allows the development of a hard and strong substructure with adequate shock protection on its outer surface.

In 1993, Inturregui *et al.* investigated the production of tension in the master metallic structure when it was screwed and tightened with 10 Ncm on plaster models obtained by three transfer molding techniques for osseointegratable oral implants. Only two implants were used to simplify the types of force produced. A master metal structure was cast in a silver-palladium alloy. The structure consisted of two gold cylinders connected by a 30 mm long bar. Two tin replicas associated with the guide pins were tightened with 10 Ncm on the metal structure. This structure was fixed to an improved stone plaster base. A total of thirty individual acrylic resin trays with an occlusal window were made (ten for each technique). The impression material used was polyether (Impregum). The guide pins were tightened with 10 Ncm. The molds were separated from the master model 6 minutes after positioning the tray. Three different techniques were used: I - unbonded square transfers; II - square transfers bonded with impression plaster; III - square transfers bonded with Duralay acrylic resin. For technique III, a polyvinylsiloxane mould (putty consistency) was constructed to standardize the spline. The spline was sectioned with a carborundum disk. The segments were re-seated on the master model, re-tightened with a torque of 10 Ncm and re-joined with acrylic resin. The acrylic resin polymerized for 15 minutes before the impression was taken. The guide pin, transfer pin and abutment analog were tightened using digital pressure only. The force of 10 Ncm applied with the torque wrench caused the transfers to rotate in the polyether molds (technique I). Therefore, digital pressure was used to tighten the brass ananglasts for all molding techniques. The molds were cast in sets of five, within a time period of less than 3½ hours from the first and at least 30 minutes from the last impression that was taken. The models obtained with improved V-type stone plaster (Die-Keen) were manually spatulated for 30 seconds and vacuum spatulated for a further 30 seconds. After a minimum of 2 hours, they were separated from the mold and stored at room temperature for 2 weeks until measurements were taken. The metal structure was screwed in place with gold screws and tightened with 10 Ncm on each plaster model obtained. Measurements in the horizontal and vertical planes were made using a digital tension indicator model P-3500 (Measurements Group Inc.). Technique I was statistically different from techniques II and III in both planes (horizontal and vertical).

In addition, technique I proved to provide values closer to those found in the master model. The authors concluded that there was a statistically significant difference between the three techniques used. None of the impression techniques resulted in an absolutely passive fit of the structure. Based on the stress values recorded and the subjective fit of the framework on the models, any of the impression techniques investigated should be clinically acceptable. It seems to be of no clinical advantage to use the more time-consuming transfer impression techniques with splinting made with self-curing acrylic resin or plaster.

Assif *et al.* (1994) suggested a molding technique for osseointegral implants that bonds the transfers directly to the individual acrylic resin tray, avoiding the use of self-curing resin and dental floss, reducing distortion and simplifying clinical procedures. An initial impression with the cylindrical transfers connected to the implants was taken with irreversible hydrocolloid and the plaster was poured. At least 48 hours before the impression, an individual tray was made with appropriate relief and perforations for the square transfers to extend beyond the top surface of the tray. A new impression was taken to construct the working model, using elastomeric material, using the injection technique around the transfers. The excess impression material was removed until it was level with the tray. A self-curing resin was applied around the square transfers, bonding them to the tray. After polymerization, the tray was removed, the analogues adapted and the final working model was cast. The splinted section containing the transfers was separated from the tray with a cutter, obtaining an index to check the accuracy of the working model. The impression technique presented allowed for easy manipulation, reduced clinical working time and minimized the distortion of the resin splint through the prior construction of the individual tray and the incremental addition technique.

Waskewicz *et al. (*1994) wrote that the primary objective in the manufacture of superstructures for osseointegrated implants is to achieve a passive fit of the connection between the abutment and the metal structure, as mechanical stress can be transmitted to the implants through the connection of the structure to the abutments. Passive fit of the abutment to the metal structure is often difficult to obtain and interpret during clinical testing. Welding techniques to correct structural discrepancies have been described. These involve either casting in separate units or sectioning in separate units and registering (joining) in the mouth or on the master model. Because of the lack of knowledge of biological responses to stress transfer, the aim of prosthodontists should be to deliver the adjusted structure as passively as possible. For this study, a photoelastic analysis was carried out to evaluate the stress patterns generated around implants with passively and non-passively adjusted metal frameworks. Five Branemark implants were positioned in a photoelastic analog of a human mandible. Visual examination of the metal framework showed an inadequate fit (a gap between the framework and abutments 4 and 5) when a gold screw was tightened in abutment 1 with a torque of 10 Ncm and vice versa. The structures were analyzed by taking photographs of the bangs resulting from the stress that was generated when the structure was screwed to the abutments with the gold screws at a torque of 10 Ncm. The non-passive structure was photoelastically analyzed by screwing it with gold screws at a torque of 10 Ncm for three different sequences: abutment 1,2,3,4,5; abutment 5,4,3,2,1; abutment 3,2,4,1,5. After an initial assessment and registration had been carried out, the non-passive structure was sectioned between each abutment for registration (joining) for welding. The gold screws were tightened to a torque of 10 Ncm, and the metal sections were joined with Duralay, encapsulated and welded. Only the sectioned and welded structure showed any stress bangs around the implants when it was tightened using the three different sequences described above. The sectioning, joining and welding of metal structures is therefore highly recommended. The sequence of screwing the framework to the abutments was insignificant, as identical stress distributions were seen with the three different tightening methods.

Kallus & Bessing (1994) evaluated the occurrence of loosening of gold and intermediate screws five years after the installation of full-arch prostheses in 50 patients (16 in the maxilla and 34 in the mandible). After connecting the abutments, 32 patients had six implants, 14 patients had five, and 4 had four implants. The prostheses made of type 3 gold, with acrylic resin teeth and using Branemark system components, had the gold screws manually tightened with maximum force in a standardized sequence. The results were related to clinical parameters such as the accuracy of the superstructure, operator dependence and clinical and radiographic diagnosis of the state of the implant after 5 years. The authors concluded that there appears to be a clinically significant correlation between prosthetic maladaptation and loosening of the gold screws, but the results are not entirely conclusive, since well-fitted prostheses can have loose screws and prostheses with poor adaptation can also support tight gold screws. Gold screw failures could be related to prosthesis maladaptation and considered to be operator-dependent to a certain extent, since screw tightening, clinical assessment of adaptation and adaptation itself are operator-dependent variables, which are affected by the operator's manual dexterity and muscle strength. According to the authors, the clinical and radiographic findings do not support the hypothesis that prostheses with poor adaptation could represent a long-term risk to osseointegration. It is recommended that full-arch fixed prostheses be retightened after 5 years.

Aparicio (1994) reports that in order to maintain osseointegration, it is essential for the prosthesis to fit completely passively, because the absence of periodontal ligament makes the implant unable to adapt its position to a non-passive structure. The traditional system of constructing the metal structure by casting on turned parts - called gold cylinders in the Branemark system - has been modified in such a way that these parts are joined to the metal structure by means of physical-chemical bonding. This bond is achieved by treating the metal surface with the Silicoater system and a composite resin cement using an improved cementation protocol. However, the ultimate success of this method is obviously limited by the accuracy of the impression procedures, because the cementation of the prosthetic structure on the cylinders is initially done on the working models, unscrewed and screwed into the mouth, where it will be allowed to harden. This paper presents the clinical feasibility of this new philosophy, demonstrated over a 2-year period. A total of 64 prostheses (39 maxillary and 25 mandibular) supported by 214 EsthetiCone (Nobelpharma) or angled abutments placed in 47 patients were evaluated, with an average observation period of 9 months. The results showed that it is possible to routinely obtain a metal-ceramic prosthesis with a totally passive circular fit while maintaining the possibility of recovery (reversibility), thus making post-ceramic welding unnecessary.

Phillips *et al.* (1994) reported that most studies have focused on the distortion of the master model obtained from a molding and on the differences between various transfer designs and transfer techniques. This study examined the position of the transfers within the mold prior to manufacturing the model and also compared the machining tolerances of a given system. Machining tolerances can be described as clinically acceptable distortions, i.e. those that do not induce stress on the components during placement in the mouth. The purpose of this study was to compare the accuracy of three different impression techniques currently used by dentists. These were: 1- conical transfers; 2- square transfers and 3- square transfers bonded with acrylic resin. The three-dimensional position of the transfers on the master model provided the control reference for direct comparison of the distortion or relative movement of the transfers during impression taking. Five implant analogs (Nobelpharma) were attached to a colorless thermosetting resin master model simulating an edentulous mandible. Each analog was placed with a 10-degree buccal angulation and fixed transmucosal abutments (TMA) (20 Ncm). This created a model equal to the clinical situation with implants slightly diverging from each other.

Transfers were fixed (10 Ncm) onto the master model and their three-dimensional position recorded using a measuring device with an accuracy of less than 1 µm for comparison of the transfer impressions. Impressions were taken using three different techniques with special trays manufactured to allow a minimum of 3 mm of impression material. The impression material used was Impregum (ESPE/Premier) and the acrylic resin for the splinting technique was GC Pattern resin, using dental floss to support it during placement. A total of fifteen samples were prepared using the three different techniques. The position of the transfers was measured within the molding to avoid distortions created by the expansion of the plaster setting. Statistical evaluations indicated that the distortions associated with the square transfers were significantly less than those with the conical transfers and the resin-splinted specimens fell between the two. For the conical transfer there are other variables, such as the distortion of the impression material during removal, causing permanent deformation of the material (remember that the implants are angled) and also the need for repositioning within the impression. There was no significant difference between the distortions of the conical transfers and the resin-splinted square transfers. The total absolute movement of each TMA at the interface with the implant replica ranged from 72.3 µm (±38.2 µm) for the conical transfers, 53.6 µm (±27.2 µm) for the resin-splinted square transfers and 35.5 µm (±20.7 µm) for the square transfers. The machining tolerances of the Nobelpharma components tested in this study were 31.9 µm (±14.2 µm) in the xy plane. This value was based on work previously carried out at the University of Washington. Comparing the machining tolerances measured for the implant system (31.9 µm) with the distortions in the xy plane of the square transfers (without resin), this was the only group that showed no statistical difference. The clinical significance of this study is that an impression technique should ideally take the shortest time, be easy to perform, inexpensive, comfortable for the patient and give the best results. The conical transfer meets most of these criteria, but its inherent inaccuracy limits its use. However, since the technique with resin-splinted square transfers has not shown any benefits over the resin-free square transfer, the extra time and complications

involved in the creation of the resin splint could be considered unnecessary.

Shiau *et al.* (1994) presented a modified impression technique with the aim of obtaining a more accurate master model. Using a cylindrical transfer mold and irreversible hydrocolloid, an individual resin tray is made for the square transfer technique bonded with Duralay. The square transfers are numbered, sectioned, placed in their correct positions intraorally and re-bonded with Duralay. After polymerization, the screws are loosened and the accuracy of the transfers is visually checked (This technique is carried out by tightening a guide screw on one terminal abutment and the other terminal transfer is examined for a gap between the abutment and the transfer). The splinted transfers are removed from the mouth and fitted to the abutments. A wax dam is built and plaster is poured. Only half the length of the anastomos remains inside the plaster matrix. After setting, the plaster index is finished. The splinted transfers are returned from the index to the mouth and their accuracy is checked again. The individual tray is tried in and the impression taken. The index is positioned inside the impression and the screws are tightened. Plaster is poured, checking that the space between the index and the impression is completely filled. The model is finished.

Assif *et al.* (1996) evaluated the accuracy of three implant molding techniques using a laboratory mandibular metal matrix that simulated a clinical situation with five implant analogs screwed together and bonded with epoxy resin. The three impression techniques were as follows: Group 1- square transfers bonded together with self-curing acrylic resin (Duralay); Group 2- square transfers without bonding and Group 3- square transfers bonded with Duralay resin directly to the individual acrylic resin tray. Fifteen impressions using polyether (Impregum F) were taken for each technique. The accuracy of each technique was analyzed using an extensometer, based on the seating (with a torque of 10 Ncm) of a metal superstructure (silver/palladium), previously made, on the plaster models obtained from the transfer impressions. The average results in microstrains were: Group 1: 138.06; Group 2: 293.60 and Group 3: 279.13. They found that joining the transfers together with self-curing acrylic resin proved to be significantly more precise than the other two techniques studied.

Cheshire & Hobkirk (1996) investigated *in vivo* the fit of five mandibular superstructures fabricated on Nobel Biocare implants, using a polyvinylsiloxane impression material to record discrepancies. The five patients had been wearing the prostheses for at least 8 months without any clinical problems. After sectioning the impressions, the vertical and horizontal discrepancies were analyzed in four places using a microscope. The discrepancies obtained were measured not only when the gold cylinder screws were tightened by hand to the maximum, but also when tightened with a torque wrench to the recommended value of 10 Ncm. Manual tightening produces a torque above 10 Ncm. The vertical discrepancies for the manually tightened abutments ranged from 0 µm to 63 µm, with an average of 14 µm. In the mechanically tightened group, the vertical discrepancy ranged from 0 to 130 µm, with an average of 21 µm. The horizontal discrepancies for the mechanically tightened abutments ranged from 0 to 140 µm, with an average of 31 µm, compared to an average of 46 µm and a range of 0 to 113 µm for the manually tightened abutments. An intimate fit was rarely achieved. A perfect fit occurs when the surfaces of the implant and prosthesis are aligned and contacted without the need to apply force. It was concluded that considerable discrepancies existed around the superstructures that had been judged to have clinically acceptable fit. The discrepancies were reduced in the vertical direction by manual tightening of the gold screws. Horizontal errors lead to bending of the gold screws, resulting in their early failure. Nobel Biocare has also stated that the elastic limit of the screws is around 17-18 Ncm. For this reason, 10 Ncm is recommended for tightening abutment screws. Manual tightening not only reduces the risk of screw fracture, but also seems to reduce the vertical discrepancy with inevitable stress transfer to the implant and screws.

Coelho (1997) evaluated the behavior of six silicone adhesives, a polyether, a polysulfide, a condensation silicone and an irreversible hydrocolloid, when used in a dental implant impression and position transfer technique. Using standardized individual trays and a master model made of acrylic, in which five implants were placed, five impressions were taken with each material tested, for a total of fifty impression procedures. The horizontal distances between the analogue components of the plaster models obtained from each impression were compared with the same distances from the master model, in order to determine the possible dimensional changes suffered by the impression material. *Analysis of* the data obtained showed that all the materials tested showed statistically significant dimensional changes. The silicone adhesive President showed the least dimensional change, while the irreversible hydrocolloid Orthoprint showed the greatest change. Finally, all the silicone adhesives produced similar models, followed by polyether, polysulphide, condensation silicone and irreversible hydrocolloid.

In 1997, Bindra & Heath evaluated the bond strength of the adhesive for trays made of two silicone adhesives (Provil and Express) and a polyether (Impregum). They used brass metal trays, self-curing acrylic resin trays and light-curing resin trays. The pairs of plates (clinically the trays) measured 45 X 45 mm each and were separated (by a jig) by 3 mm to ensure a uniform thickness of the molding material. The surfaces of the plates were cleaned with chloroform. To remove adhesive residue from previous impressions, the resin plates were sanded to a grit of 150. The adhesive was applied for 1 min and left to dry at 23°C for 15 min. After applying the impression material, it was left to set in an oven at 37°C with 100% humidity. They concluded that the use of adhesive was significant for

Provil and Express, but not for Impregum. Provil adhesive can be used on Expess and vice versa (Provil adhesive is even better). The failure of the silicones occurred at the adhesive-molding material interface, with adhesive remaining in the "tray". With Impregum, most of the failures occurred at the adhesive-"tray" interface (it is therefore advisable to use perforated or sprayed trays). Some specimens with Impregum showed cohesive failure. Provil and Express adhered most strongly to brass trays, while the combination of Impregum and light-curing resin trays provided the strongest bond. In fact, light-curing resin trays provided greater adhesion than acrylic resin trays. No correlation was established between the speed of separation during the tests and bond strength. Based on the results obtained, the authors conclude that the application of adhesive results in a significant increase in the bond between impression material and tray.

Burawi *et al.* (1997) evaluated the accuracy of the splinted and non-splinted impression technique. On a type IV plaster master model with five implants, a metallic gold structure was built on gold cylinders. As it was poorly adapted, it was sectioned between the abutments and joined with cyanoacrylate for welding. Markings were made on the metal structure and it was sectioned again at four points with a 0.45 mm thick diamond blade. Thirty individual impression trays (3 mm thick) made of acrylic resin with perforations and openings in the region of the abutments were used to take the impressions. Three localizing depressions were made on the model to standardize the positioning of the tray during the impressions. Adhesive was applied internally and extended 2 mm externally to the tray. It was left to dry for 15 minutes. The impressions were taken with silicone adhesive (Elite) using the one-step technique. The light material was injected with an automatic mixing syringe around the abutments and immediately the tray with the heavy material was seated until the stops contacted the base of the master model. We waited 15 minutes from the start of mixing (twice the manufacturer's recommendation to compensate for polymerization at room temperature). The unpainted technique used was as follows: the plastic transfers had internally and externally anti-rotational locator schemes. They were removed along with the impression. The metal transfers were unscrewed from the abutments of the master model and fixed with connecting screws to the laboratory analogues. Each assembled set of metal transfer and analog was then pressed into the position marked with guides on the plastic transfer inside the impression. The splinting technique used was as follows: 24 hours before the impression, a splint was made with dental floss and Duralay. Cuts were made to leave a 2 mm gap between each pair of transfers 15 minutes before the impression was taken, and the acrylic resin sections of the splinting were bonded with Duralay. The same acrylic resin splint was used to transfer the impression components from the master model to all 15 analogue models made with the splinting technique. Where necessary, the splint was sectioned and grouted as described above. The connecting screws were tightened by hand. The seating surfaces of all components were cleaned with isopropyl alcohol before each connection procedure for all techniques. All molds were kept at room temperature (25° C) for 1 hour. The plaster was proportioned, mixed manually for 15 seconds to incorporate the water and then mechanically mixed under vacuum for 30 seconds. Waiting 1 hour before separating the molding. The metal frame segments were tightened in each of the thirty models with a constant torque of 10 Ncm. A measuring microscope with an accuracy of 0.001 mm was used to take readings of the distances between the lines marked on the framework. The authors concluded that the greatest errors occurred in the anteroposterior horizontal plane for the splinted technique (0.26 to 0.85 mm). Errors of this magnitude could certainly prevent the precise seating of the metal structure, necessitating its sectioning and welding. In the mesiodistal horizontal plane, both techniques reproduced these dimensions with minimal and perhaps clinically tolerable error (0.021 to 0.052 mm). The errors in the vertical plane appeared to be similar in both techniques (0.0006 to 0.134 mm), requiring corrective measures in some situations.

In 1997, Hussaini & Wong presented a clinical and laboratory procedure for making a precise working model that will facilitate the fabrication of the casting on the master model. The square transfers are joined in the mouth with acrylic resin (GC pattern resin) and dental floss. The assembly is unscrewed and sectioned with a thin disk. It is placed back in the mouth and the spaces created are joined with acrylic resin or light-curing composite resin. The molding is done with polyvinylsiloxane using an open tray to access the screws. Using a brush or cement spatula, the apical portion of the ananglasts is firmly bonded with impression plaster (setting expansion of 0.06%). After the plaster has set, each interproximal space is sectioned with a thin disk. Soak for a few minutes in plaster water and rinse. The separated parts are then rejoined with a second plaster mixture for impression taking. At this point, the impression is dyed and soft tissue material is poured around the coronal end of the ankles and the impression is poured with type III plaster (0.3% setting expansion). One model was made using this technique and another was made using type III plaster without the impression plaster procedure. In the model made using the proposed procedure, the gaps between the implant head and the prosthetic structure (measured with an optical microscope) ranged from 20 to 36 µm, whereas in the conventional model the gaps ranged from 82 to 139 µm. When a precise working model is made, the dentist can instruct the laboratory to cast each unit separately and weld them using the master model as an index. By using the proposed procedure, if the final casting fits the master model, the dentist can be confident that it will fit the patient's mouth. Although a clinical presentation is unlikely to prove the superiority of a procedure, this article exposes another method that can be used and tested in a scientific study.

In 1998, Goiato *et al.* reported that, for many edentulous patients, the use of osseointegrated implants in the remaining alveolar ridge has been indicated, with the aim of increasing the retention and stability of the total prosthesis. However, one of the reasons for the failure of a total prosthesis on implants lies in the lack of precision in adapting the connection system for these prostheses. This depends on the type of impression material and the prosthetic component transfer techniques used to obtain the working model, where the impression must precisely reproduce the anatomical details and establish the transfer correctly. Thus, in the Branemark system there are square and conical transfers that lend themselves to transfers and adapt to intermediates and their replicas. However, there are different techniques for using them, resulting in research that seeks to identify the superiority of one technique over another. The purpose of this study was to verify the linear dimensional change in reproductions of the metal matrix with four osseointegratable implants, made with three impression materials and three transfer molding techniques. The molding materials were: silicone by addition (Express); silicone by condensation (Optosil- Xantopren) and polyether (Impregum F). The transfer molding techniques adopted were: square transfers adapted with Duralay resin sculpted into a square shape, in order to retain the transfers when removing them from the mold; technique with square transfers joined with Duralay resin using the dental floss technique; and technique with conical transfers. To standardize the impression pressure, a load of 1500g was placed on the tray, enough to remove the excess impression material and keep it confined at a constant pressure. The prosthetic transfers were unscrewed from the plaster models and the cylindrical reference transfers were screwed onto them, with the ends marked with a geometric center point. Measurements were made using a Carl Zeiss comparator microscope. All the impression materials reproduced the matrix reference points, with values that were not statistically significant, in all the transfer techniques, except for Optosil-Xantopren in the square transfer technique and the conical transfer technique. The transfer technique bonded with Duralay acrylic resin showed no statistically significant difference, suggesting stable linear conditions in all three types of elastomeric impression materials. All transfer techniques produced linear dimensional changes in the models without statistically significant differences, regardless of the impression materials.

Assif *et al.* (1999) evaluated the accuracy of three implant molding techniques, using three different transfer bonding materials. They used a laboratory metal matrix with five implants that simulated clinical practice. For group A, a self-curing acrylic resin (Duralay, Reliance) was used. In group B, a dual-curing acrylic resin (Accuset, EDS) was used and in group C, impression plaster (Kerr Snow White Plaster n° 2, Kerr USA) was used, which was also the impression material in this group. A metal superstructure with passive implant seating was built on top of the matrix, and this was used to check the accuracy of the position of the implant analogs in the replicas. For groups A and B, polyether (Impregum F) was used as the impression material. Fifteen impressions were taken for each group. The accuracy of the plaster models with the implant analogs was measured by adapting the superstructure to them, using a strain gauge. Statistical analysis revealed that there was a significant difference between groups A and B and between groups B and C, but no significant difference between groups A and C. They concluded that impression techniques using self-curing acrylic resin or impression plaster as the transfer bonding material were significantly more precise than when using double-curing acrylic resin. This may be caused by the incomplete polymerization of the double-cured acrylic resin and it may also be that the contraction during polymerization generates stresses in the transfer/acrylic resin interface. The authors recommended plaster as the material of choice for implant transfer molding in completely edentulous patients (and without any anatomical limitations such as bone retention), as it hardens quickly, is completely accurate and rigid, does not flex or deform, is easy to manipulate, is less time-consuming and is more affordable.

In 1999, Gregory *et al.* described a procedure that allows careful edge correction and shaping of an edentulous arch, simultaneously with the transfer of implant shaping components. The resulting master model is accurate in terms of soft tissue details, implant component positioning and the relationship between soft tissue and implants. The first step is a conventional edge impression and full impression with an individual tray. Once the impression has been removed from the mouth, the transfers are placed over the implants. Openings are made in the tray wide enough to allow it to sit in the mouth without touching the transfers. When the impression has settled completely and passively, a self-curing acrylic resin or light-curing resin is injected around the transfers. After the resin has polymerized, the screws and the impression are removed. The ananglasts are placed on the transfers and the master model is fabricated using conventional means. The procedure described in this article focuses on several significant problems with implant-supported overdenture molding. The distance between the abutments in overdentures makes it difficult to splint the transfers in the mouth with conventional techniques (floss mesh and self-curing acrylic resin). However, there are some disadvantages to this two-step procedure: as a result of the holes in the tray, some impression detail may be lost around the transfers, but as the bar and abutment will be relieved before processing the denture, this will not affect the fit of the *overdenture.* Another disadvantage is the extra clinical time required to drill the holes in the tray and splint with resin intraorally.

Dumbrigue *et al.* (2000) attested that bonding the transfers with acrylic resin during the impression procedures increases the accuracy of transferring the spatial relationship of the implants to the master model. However, distortions can occur during the splinting procedure due to the polymerization contraction of the resin. They recommended the use of acrylic resin bars between the transfers so that the amount of resin to be polymerized is small, thus minimizing this effect. These bars are made with GC Pattern Resin injected into 3 mm diameter straws. After at least 17 minutes, the resin bar is released from the straw and should only be used after 24 hours (because the full contraction of 6.5 to 7.9% occurs within 24 hours). The resin bar is sectioned into appropriate lengths to close the space between adjacent transfers. Using the brush technique, the ends of the resin bars are bonded to the transfers with acrylic resin. The applied resin must be allowed to harden for at least 17 minutes before the final impression is taken (because 80% of resin contraction occurs in the first 17 minutes after mixing). The final impression is taken using an individual tray and the impression material of choice.

Herbst *et al.* (2000) evaluated and compared four molding techniques in terms of their dimensional accuracy for reproducing the position of implants in working models. A metal matrix was constructed with five implants positioned to simulate a clinical situation, two of which had an 8° lingual inclination and eight reference points milled into the metal matrix. Four molding techniques were used: (1) conical transfers, (2) square transfers, (3) square transfers bonded with self-curing acrylic resin (Duralay) and (4) square transfers with lateral metal extension on one side (unsplinted), which only rested against the adjacent transfer (Southern Implants, South Africa). A torque of 10 Ncm was applied to standardize the fit of each healing cap (with a reference point on its surface) over each analogue on the master model or plaster models. The bonding with Duralay acrylic resin and dental floss was done 20 min before the impression was taken to allow optimum polymerization and match the clinical situation. The master model was kept in an oven with 100% humidity and at 37° C while the impressions were taken. The impressions were made with silicone by mass/regular addition (President - Coltene), using the simultaneous impression technique with individual self-curing acrylic resin trays (Formatray - Kerr). Four models were made for each technique and kept at room temperature for at least 24 hours before measurements. The plaster specimens (Vel Mix - Dentsply) were analyzed using a reflective light microscope capable of analyzing the x, y and z axes. They observed that dimensional accuracy was high and, although statistically significant, a maximum distortion difference of only 0.31% was recorded. They concluded that the dimensional accuracy of all the techniques evaluated was exceptional and the differences observed can be considered to be clinically negligible, therefore all of them are recommended for transfer molding of osseointegrated implants. One clinical implication of these results is that it does not seem to be clinically advantageous to bond the transfers with self-curing acrylic resin.

Lorenzoni *et al.* (2000) stated that accurate transfer of the implant position to the model is a prerequisite for passive seating of the suprastructure and that inaccurate structures result in stress between the components and at the implant-bone interface. The authors compared three impression materials (polyether - Impregum F regular with individual acrylic resin tray; Polyvinylsiloxane - heavy/light with one-step technique and reversible hydrocolloid) using the Frialit® -2 implant system and the indirect technique. A model with eight Frialit implant analogs was used. Four abutments on the right side received acrylic resin transfers (TC) and the four abutments on the left were left without TC? The use of TCs to improve transfer accuracy was tested with all three materials. Six impressions of the original model were taken for each of the three materials. In order to compensate for the delay in polymerization time at room temperature, the elastomeric materials were given 12 minutes from the start of mixing. The molds were cast with GC Fujirock plaster. The readings were taken on a 3D machine capable of locating points in space and calculating the relative distortion of the tilt angles (rot-XY, rot-XZ, rot-YZ) and the three-dimensional displacement. The results suggest that silicon adhesive and polyether are the materials of choice for transfer molding procedures for implants. The use of transfers resulted in a significant reduction in rotation in the XY plane, but did not improve absolute three-dimensional displacement. Silicone by addition with the use of transfer agents proved to be very accurate. The comparison between polyether and addition silicon showed a significant difference in xy rotation and three-dimensional displacement in favor of silicon. Because the average distortions between the matrix and the replicas were approximately 100 μm, absolutely precise seating may not be achieved due to the physical properties of the materials. The authors also stressed the need for studies to assess the amount of stress tolerable at the implant/bone interface.

Nissan *et al.* (2000) evaluated the accuracy of three heavy-light impression techniques using the same impression material (polyvinylsiloxane) in a laboratory model. The three heavy-light molding techniques used were: (1) One step (heavy and light molding materials used simultaneously); (2) Two steps, with 2 mm of relief obtained with prefabricated transfers (the heavy material is used first as a preliminary molding to create 2 mm of space for the light material); and (3) two-step technique, with a polyethylene spacer (plastic spacer used in the molding with the heavy material first and then the next phase is carried out with the light material). For each technique, fifteen impressions were taken of a stainless steel master model containing three full crown preparations, which was used as a positive control. Accuracy was assessed by measuring six dimensions (intra-abutment and inter-abutment) on the dies obtained from the master model impressions. Statistically significant differences were observed between the three impression techniques for all intra-abutment and inter-abutment measurements. Overall discrepancies in the two-step technique with 2 mm of relief were significantly lower than in the one-step or two-step impression techniques with a polyethylene spacer. The two-step molding technique with 2 mm of relief was the most accurate for fabricating plaster dies.

Vigolo *et al.* (2000) evaluated *in vitro* the accuracy of models obtained from transfer impressions using square transfers to replace a single tooth. The transfers were divided into two groups, with the first group using the transfers as supplied by the manufacturer and the second group receiving sandblasting (50 μm aluminum oxide at a pressure of 2.5 atmospheres) followed by the application of tray adhesive. A resin model with a single implant located in the region of the upper right 2nd premolar was used to simulate a clinical situation. Before each impression procedure, the square transfer was screwed onto the implant of the resin model using a torque wrench calibrated to 10 Ncm. The transfer molds were made with polyether (Impregum - Espe) spatulated in a mechanical spatulator (Pentamix, ESPE) for the two groups studied. The Impregum adhesive was applied to each individual resin tray (Palatray LC, Kulzer Heraeus) 1 hour before the impressions were taken. Twenty impressions were taken for each group. Twenty-four hours after the impression was taken, the implant replica was screwed onto the protractor and the impression was poured with type IV stone plaster (New Fujirock, GC). The models obtained were analyzed using a profilometer (Nikon model V-12) to check for possible changes in the position (rotation) of the hexagon of the implant replicas in the plaster models, compared to the resin model. They observed that the change in the position of the hexagon in the replicas was significantly less in the models obtained with the modified transfers than with the unprepared transfers. They concluded that the accuracy of transfer moulding increases when the transfers are sprayed and covered with the adhesive of the moulding material.

Romero *et al.* (2000) evaluated 3 post-casting techniques to correct non-passive fit between a cast bar superstructure and its interface with an implant abutment. A metal model consisting of two titanium PME HL 3.8/4.5 abutments was used in this study. Thirty pre-fabricated implant bars of 18 mm in length were used to make the metal structures. Initial measurements were taken on the y-axis of the interface between the bar and the left abutment using a microscope. Averages of the buccal, distal and lingual measurements of each specimen were calculated. Ten specimens were sectioned, indexed and repaired by casting in the same metal alloy (group 1). Ten specimens were sectioned, indexed and repaired with welding (Group 2). The last ten specimens were subjected to two cycles of *electrical discharge machining on the MedArc M-2 EDM machine (Group 3).* Post-repair measurements were taken from all three groups. The initial mean crack widths were 192 µm for Group 1, 190 µm for Group 2 and 198 µm for Group 3. There was a significant difference in the mean number of cracks between group 1 (15 µm) and group 2 (72 µm) and also between groups 2 (72 µm) and 3 (7.5 µm) after each repair technique. No difference could be detected between groups 1 and 3. The group subjected to electrical discharge machining resulted in the smallest average crack (7.5 µm), following the criteria described in the literature for passive seating (up to 10 µm).

Wee (2000) evaluated the amount of torque required to rotate the square transfers in various impression materials while tightening the abutment replicas and compared the accuracy of the models obtained from the transfer impression procedures using the direct technique with different impression materials. The master model was a metal matrix with five stainless steel abutment replicas 12 mm apart. The purpose of this study was not to evaluate the abutment-metal framework relationship. This study only evaluated the distortion of the translational resultant (x, y and z axes) of the abutment replicas from one to the other. The molding materials used were: polyether (Impregum), silicone by addition (Extrude), silicone by condensation (Elasticon) and polysulfide (Permlastic), all with different viscosities. The lack of detectable torque when using combinations of high/medium or high/low consistencies shows no advantage in using them for implant molding by the direct technique. The design of most transfers is not complicated enough to require a low consistency impression material to be injected around them. The square transfers were manually clamped into the metal matrix. Thirty impressions of the master model were made, ten for each of the three impression materials that had detectable torque values: medium viscosity polyether; high viscosity silicone adhesive; and medium viscosity polysulphide. The torque at the moment of turning the transfer inside the mold was calculated using a device called Compudriver. The accuracy of the transfers was checked by measuring the linear distances between the reference components (steel balls) fitted to each analog using a comparator microscope. The highest torque was required to rotate the protractor in the medium-viscosity polyether mold (141.3×10^{-3} mN), followed by high-viscosity silicone (71×10^{-3} mN), while for polysulfide a lower torque (51.5×10^{-3} mN) was sufficient to rotate the protractor. The models obtained from impressions with medium-viscosity polyether (average distortion of 16.2 µm) or high-viscosity adhesive silicon (15.2 µm) were significantly more accurate than polysulphide (26.2 µm) and are recommended for transfer impressions in implantology. From a clinical point of view, the results of this study support the use of polyether for multiple implant impressions in edentulous patients. The rigidity of polyether provides resistance to accidental displacement of the transfers in implant impressions. However, using polyether for an impression of a partially edentulous arch also increases the difficulty of removing the intraoral impression. High-consistency silicone adhesives and medium-consistency polysulphide are viable alternative materials of choice for experienced dentists. Silicone adhesive with its more favorable modulus of elasticity allows for easy removal of the impression.

Daoudi *et al.* (2001) in a laboratory study investigated the accuracy of four implant casting procedures using two casting techniques and two different materials. An acrylic resin maxillary master model with an implant replacing the right central incisor was used to produce forty different plaster models incorporating laboratory implants or abutment analogues in different combinations of the two impression techniques (the implant-level transfer repositioning technique and the direct abutment-level CeraOne - plastic transfer technique) and materials (President - polyvinylsiloxane and Impregum F - polyether). The results showed greater variations in the position of the analog with the repositioning impression technique (conical transfer - indirect technique) than with the direct technique. The anteroposterior error for the repositioning technique was more than twice that of the direct technique. The rotational errors in the repositioning technique were large enough to be of clinical concern. No significant difference was found between the polyvinylsiloxane and polyether impression materials for the two types of impression techniques tested. The authors concluded that the repositioning impression technique may produce less predictable results than the direct technique and that the choice of impression material made no significant difference.

Pinto *et al.* (2001) compared three molding techniques on a standard polyethylene model simulating an edentulous mandible with three implants. The impressions were made with polysulphide using an individual acrylic resin tray with an upper opening in the implant region to provide access to the square impression components of groups II and III (bonded with Duralay). For the impressions with the conical components (group I), the tray opening was closed with wax to prevent the impression material from leaking out. The tray was fitted with locators so that it could always be positioned in the same position on the standard model. Ten molds were obtained for each group, and during molding, the trays received a constant pressure of 400g for 20 minutes. The molds were immediately poured with type IV plaster (Vel-mix) and separated after two hours. The plaster models were measured using a profilometer (Starret Sigma VB 300, North Yorkshire), measuring the distances between the internal edges of each replica to compare with the originals (made on the standard model). As with the standard model, each reading was repeated three times and the arithmetic mean corresponded to the horizontal distance between the replicas. Although there was no statistically significant difference between the horizontal measurements of the three groups, which means that the three techniques provided similar models in the dimensions analyzed, when these measurements were compared with those of the standard model, statistically significant differences were observed (with the plaster models showing greater horizontal distances than the originals). Based on the results of this study, it is to be expected that the sequence of procedures for obtaining infrastructures for fixed prostheses carried out on models obtained by any of these three techniques would result in undue pressure or poor adaptation, making it difficult to obtain the desired passive adaptation. For this reason, it seems obvious that welding the parts together or dividing the prostheses using semi-precision fittings are methods that would reduce the incidence of stresses at the prosthesis/implant/bone interface.

Sahin & Çehreli (2001) review the clinical significance of passive fit and the factors that affect the final fit of implant-supported structures. One of the main challenges for a prosthodontist is to deliver an acceptable prosthesis that does not compromise the longevity of the treatment. Passive fit (synonymous with "ideal fit") is assumed to be one of the most significant prerequisites for maintaining the bone-implant interface. To provide passive fit or a stress-free superstructure, the structure should theoretically induce absolutely zero stress on the implant components and the surrounding bone in the absence of an applied external load. This vital requirement can be provided by complete and simultaneous contact of the inner surfaces of all retainers by all abutments. A structure with an absolutely passive fit has not been achieved in the last three decades.

Although there is no consensus, there are various suggestions regarding the acceptable level of misfit. Taking into account current knowledge, although there are claims that passive fit is a governing factor for maintaining osseointegration and implant success, there is a growing contrary trend in the relevant literature. The laboratory and clinical procedures used to fabricate frameworks are inadequate to provide an absolutely passive fit for implant-supported fixed superstructures and require further research and development. Achieving a passive fit does not appear to be possible and may in fact be unnecessary (although some prosthetic complications are attributed to the lack of a passive fit, its effect on implant success is questionable).

Wise (2001) comments that the impression and model on which an implant-supported fixed prosthesis is fabricated must accurately reproduce the intraoral relationship. The fit of fixed prostheses fabricated on master models cast in improved type IV stone plaster (Vel-Mix, Kerr - setting expansion of 0.08%) and in a low-expansion molding plaster (Gnathostone, Zeus - setting expansion of 0.02%) was investigated *in vitro*. An impression was taken of each of the replicas of patients with implant-abutment distances of 50 and 35 mm, using square transfers and impression plaster. As it is a rigid material, the impression plaster reduced the possibility of the torque used to tighten the abutment replica inside the transfer causing it to move inside the mold. For each of the impressions, ten master models were cast with Velmix plaster and ten with Gnathostone. A "simulated fixed prosthesis" in impression plaster was fabricated on each master model and then returned in a random order to the appropriate patient replica. The fixed prostheses were screwed onto an abutment with a torque of 10 Ncm. Vertical discrepancies were measured on the other abutment (by projecting the slides made with a Nikon F-90X camera with a Micro Nikkor 50 mm macro lens at 50x magnification). For an inter-pillar distance of 50 mm, Velmix plaster models produced an average vertical discrepancy of 80 µm (standard deviation = 32.50 µm and range 36.7 to 153.3 µm). Models with low-expansion plaster produced an average vertical discrepancy of 42.8 µm (standard deviation = 12.17 µm and range 20 to 60 µm). The means were significantly different (P = 0.01). For the 35 mm inter-pillar distance, the average vertical discrepancies produced by Vel-Mix plaster and low-expansion plaster were 84.33 µm (standard deviation = 49.9 µm and range 0 to 153.3 µm) and 0 µm (standard deviation = 0) respectively. The means were significantly different (P <0.001). A significant difference was found between the means of the vertical discrepancies of fixed prostheses produced from low-expansion plaster models with inter-pillar distances of 50 mm and low-expansion plaster models with inter-pillar distances of 35 mm (P = 0.003). No significant difference was found between the mean vertical discrepancies for fixed prostheses fabricated on improved stone plaster models (Vel-Mix). In this *in vitro* study, models cast with low-expansion plaster limited to an inter-abutment dimension of no more than 35 mm were more accurate than models with inter-abutment distances of 50 mm or than those cast with improved stone plaster (Vel-Mix). *Notes:* (1) Because of the lower compressive strength of impression plaster when compared to improved stone plaster (Gnathostone = 610 kg/cm^2 , Velmix = 840 kg/cm^2) and because of the difficulty in vacuum spatulating impression plaster, it is recommended that master dies for prepared teeth should not be cast in this material; (2) When the fixed prostheses made of impression plaster were repositioned on their respective master models, thirty-seven of the forty prostheses had a discrepancy of 0 µm and three had a discrepancy of 10 µm, demonstrating the excellent quality of the impression plaster for joining the transfers.

Ness *et al.* (1992) conducted an *in vitro* study to determine the precision of the fit to the implant abutments of three acrylic resins when used to make frameworks for implant-supported prostheses (Relate - Parkell, a vinylmethacrylate; GC Pattern Resin - GC, a polymethylmethacrylate; Duralay - Loctite, a polymethylmethacrylate). For this analysis, they built a master model in Ivovap acrylic resin (Ivoclar) containing five Nobelpharma titanium implants. Using this model, five standardized arch-shaped acrylic resin structures were fabricated for each acrylic resin tested. Duralay was the most fluid and allowed easy injection. GC was the most viscous and had the fastest initial setting time. The fabricated patterns remained in the master model for 24 hours before being removed and subsequently measured (taking readings in three directions x, y, z). Measurements were made before the patterns were fabricated, with the gold cylinders on their respective pillars, and after the fabrication of the patterns, when the patterns had been removed from the master model. The results of this study showed that there was a significant difference in accuracy between the acrylic resins tested and that none of them was completely accurate. Decreasing the width of the arch or displacement in the x-axis and decreasing the length of the arch or displacement in the y-direction could cause misalignment of the gold cylinder with its abutment in the horizontal plane. Clinically this could look like a horizontal step between the gold cylinder and the abutment or displacement in the z-axis could cause both a vertical crack and premature contact between a cylinder and its abutment. Both GC and Duralay exhibited a lowering of the bow end whereas Relate exhibited a lifting of the bow end. From the point of view of fitting the pattern to the patient, the distortions of decreasing arch length and width and deflection at the end of the arch are only part of the need for precision. If the machining tolerance between the gold cylinder and its abutment allows a lateral movement (x or y) greater than the computed displacements, then these displacements may not be significant. Any displacement in the z-axis, however, imposes a load that forces the cylinders into contact with the pillars. In structures made with Duralay or GC resin, the end cylinders must be pulled upwards and the central cylinders pulled downwards to achieve contact with the pillars. The manufacture of a resin monoblock structure was shown to induce distortions which, if duplicated (or increased) in the casting of the metal structure, could lead to a pre-load in the structure-implant system. They concluded that all three resins suffered distortions (caused displacement of the gold cylinders) under the conditions tested. When the decreases in arch width were analyzed, the GC and Relate resins produced significantly smaller displacements than those produced by the Duralay resin. Decreases in length were only significant for Relate. Goiato *et al.* (2002) reported that for many edentulous patients, the indication of osseointegratable implants are solutions found today to increase the retention and stability of Total Prosthesis. The adaptation of the connection system of these prostheses depends on the type of impression material and the transfer techniques. The purpose of this study was to verify the dimensional change in the reproduction of a matrix with two implants, with a soft base simulating the mucosa, made with three impression materials (Lysanda zinc eugenol paste, Impregum F polyether and Jeltrate alginate) and 3 transfer techniques (conical, square and square transfers joined with dental floss covered with Duralay resin). They commented that when conical transfers are repositioned inside the mold, they can be positioned incorrectly, as well as during vibration when filling the plaster. The results were as follows: (1) all the molding materials and transfer techniques showed dimensional changes between themselves; (2) alginate showed a statistically significant difference between the other materials, with the exception of the technique with the joined square, and also showed a statistically significant difference between themselves and the transfer molding techniques; (3) the molding materials polyether and zinc oxide and eugenol paste showed no statistically significant difference between themselves and in relation to the molding techniques.

Nissan *et al.* (2002) stated that variations in relief in the heavy-light impression technique can result in dimensional changes proportional to the thickness of the light material. The purpose of this study was to determine the amount of relief required to obtain accurate plaster models using the two-step impression technique using polyvinylsiloxane impression material (President-Plus). A total of forty-five impressions were taken of a stainless steel master model, fifteen impressions for each thickness of the lightweight material (1, 2 and 3 mm). The model contained three full crown preparations which were used as the positive control. A perforated metal tray brushed with the adhesive supplied by the manufacturer was used. The laboratory steps performed were: Molding with the heavy material and waiting 10 minutes. Removal of the relieving agents, molding with the light adhesive and waiting 12 minutes (the setting time recommended by the manufacturer was doubled to compensate for the molding done at room temperature of 25° C instead of oral temperature). All impressions were stored at room temperature of 25° C for 1 hour before pouring. Improved stone plaster was spatulated manually to incorporate water and then mechanically mixed under vacuum for 15s. A vibrator was used during pouring and 1 hour was waited before separating the model. Each specimen was measured three times. The master model was measured ten times. Accuracy was assessed by measuring six dimensions (occlusogingival and inter-abutment) on the dies obtained from the master model casts. Changes in the vertical (occlusogingival) dimensions were greater than the horizontal (inter-abutment) ones. This phenomenon occurred due to the molding material contracting towards the walls of the tray, making the plaster model wider horizontally and shorter vertically. Statistically significant differences were observed between the three light material thickness groups for all occlusogingival and inter-abutment measurements. The overall discrepancies of the groups using thicknesses of 1 and 2 mm were smaller than the group with a thickness of 3 mm. Therefore, thicknesses of 1 and 2 mm of the lightweight material were much more accurate for fabricating dies. This can be achieved by using the temporary crown to create the desired space for the light material during the preliminary molding with the heavy material. Thicknesses greater than 2 mm were unsuitable for obtaining precise dies.

Nissan *et al.* (July 2002) described an implant impression technique for partially edentulous patients in which impression plaster and irreversible hydrocolloid are used. The technique ensures accuracy, ease of manipulation and reduced working time. Impression plaster is used to splint the transfers and make an impression of the implant-supported fixed partial denture. The rest of the dental arch is molded with irreversible hydrocolloid. An individual split tray incorporates both impression materials. The implant area is limited by separating the acrylic partitions and access holes are drilled on the transfers to allow easy and precise adaptation of the loaded tray and removal of the screws. The tray is loaded simultaneously with impression plaster (Snow-White paster No. 2; Kerr USA, Romulus, Mich.) in the confined area of the implants and with irreversible hydrocolloid in the rest of the split tray. It is positioned correctly in the patient's mouth and the two impression materials are allowed to set. The tray is removed, the implant rings are connected and the final working model can be cast.

De La Cruz *et al.* (2002) commented that implant verification jigs are commonly used during the manufacture of implant-supported prostheses and the dimensional accuracy of these jigs is unknown. The authors compared the dimensional accuracy of verification jigs with that of conventional impression procedures; they measured the dimensional accuracy of three resins used to make verification jigs. Thirty verification jigs and twenty impressions were made of three Steri-Oss hexagonal implants (screwed into a machined aluminum base and fixed with epoxy resin - the abutments were torqued to 35 Ncm) according to the following groups (ten samples for each group):   Group   1-   GC   patternresin   jig (polymethylmethacrylate); Group 2- Duralay resin jig (polymethylmethacrylate); Group 3- Triadgel   res   in jig (urethane-dimethacrylate);   Group   4- Molding with closed tray transfers and Group 5- Molding with open tray transfers. A plaster base was fabricated for each experimental jig and impression. The plastic bars were cut using an extra-thin diamond disk (250 □ m thick). This allowed potential forces caused by resin contraction to be relaxed. The cut regions were joined 24 hours later. Aluminum bases and experimental plaster bases were measured using the following method: X and Y coordinates of the center of each implant were obtained with a microscope by averaging the X and Y coordinates of the corners of the external hexagon implants. The origins of the coordinates during the measurement of each base were arbitrary. The distances between the points in the center of the implants were calculated using the Pythagorean theorem. Vertical measurements (Z-plane) were taken with a digital caliper at the two end implant sites. Inter-implant distances and vertical measurements were subtracted from those of the master base and the resulting distortion values were analyzed. Verification jigs were not significantly more accurate than common impression procedures. Open tray impressions showed significantly greater vertical distortion compared to the other groups. Triad gel jigs showed significantly greater distortion at the inter-implant distance (C-L) than closed tray impressions, while Duralay jigs exhibited significantly greater distortion than closed tray impressions, open tray impressions and GC pattern resin jigs at the R-C inter-implant distance. Although there was no significant difference in the other groups, the closed tray group showed the lowest mean distortion values in all measurements. They concluded that the accuracy provided by verification jigs was not significantly superior to common impression procedures. The results suggest that jig fabrication does not improve the dimensional accuracy of plaster models.

Abdullah & Talic (2003) evaluated the tensile strength of two systems of impression materials (polysulphide and polyvinylsiloxane) for two individual tray materials (chemically activated and light-curing acrylic resin). The effect of polymerizing the tray-making materials directly against the spacer wax and tin foil was evaluated for each material. The use of tin foil over the spacer material has been recommended to prevent any wax residue remaining in the individual tray, since wax can interfere with the adhesion of elastomeric impression materials. Polymerization of tray-making materials against tin foil significantly increased the adhesive strengths of polysulphide and polyvinylsiloxane to VLC and self-curing acrylic resins. The combination of polyvinylsiloxane and VLC polymerized against tin foil produced the highest adhesions. The VLC resin tray generated greater bond strength than the self-curing acrylic resin when polymerized against tin foil.

Vigolo *et al.* (2003) reported that the movement of the transfers within the impression material during the clinical and laboratory phases can cause inaccuracies in the transfer of the spatial positioning of the implants from the oral cavity to the master model. This *in vitro* study evaluated the accuracy of three different molding techniques using medium-viscosity polyether (Impregum Penta) to obtain the models. A metallic model with six implants and a metallic structure that passively adjusted to it was manufactured. A total of forty-five impressions of this model were made using square transfer agents. Three groups with fifteen models each were formed from the different molding techniques: group 1- square transfers; group 2- square transfers bonded with Duralay acrylic resin (manufactured one day before the molding, sectioned between the transfers and bonded again before the molding procedure) and group 3- square transfers sandblasted and coated with the molding adhesive indicated by the manufacturer. The Die stone plaster models (new Fuji Rock; GC Corp, Tokyo, Japan) were fabricated using the Zeiser die-casting system (Girrbach Dental GmbH, Pforzheim, Germany) to avoid problems related to plaster setting. As the metal structure was passively adjusted to the metal model, no visually perceptible resistance or bulging was found, so it was used as a control to assess the accuracy of the passive adjustment. The positioning accuracy of the abutments was numerically assessed with a Nikon profilometer (model V-12, Nikon Corp, Nippon Kogaku, Japan) at 10 times magnification, providing an accuracy of 2 µm in relation to the horizontal distances between the two most posterior abutments and the two most anterior abutments. The data was analyzed using an analysis of variance with a classification criterion (a = 0.05), followed by the Student Newman-Keuls method (P = 0.05). Visual examination of the group 1 models revealed discrepancies between one or more pillars and the metal structure. Visual analysis of the models in groups 2 and 3 revealed perfect adaptation of the metal structure to all 6 abutments. A statistically significant difference was found between the three impression techniques (P < 0.001). The Newman-Keuls procedure found significant differences between the groups, with the models in groups 2 and 3 being significantly more accurate than the models in group 1 (P =0   .05). The distance between abutments 1 and 6 compared to the metal model was 78.16 µm (SD ± 22.14) greater in group 1 models; 33.83 µm (SD ± 5.4) greater in group 2 models and 31.72 µm (SD ± 4.6) greater in group 3 models. The distances between the most anterior abutments were also greater than those recorded in the metal model. The distance was 67.91 µm (SD ± 15.34) greater in group 1 models; 31.42 µm (SD ± 7.6) greater in group 2 models and 30.34 µm (SD ± 6.4) greater in group 3 models. Within the limitations of this study, the most accurate models were obtained from the molding techniques with the square transfers bonded with Duralay acrylic resin (group 2) or with the square transfers sandblasted and covered with adhesive (group 3).

Assunçâo *et al.* (2004) evaluated the accuracy of the transfer process under varying conditions in relation to the angles of the implant anangles, materials and printing techniques. Sixty replicas of a metal matrix (control) containing four implants at 90, 80, 75 and 65 degrees to the horizontal surface were obtained using three printing techniques: T1 - indirect technique with conical transfers in closed trays; T2 - direct technique with square transfers in open trays; and T3 - square transfers bonded with self-curing acrylic resin and 4 elastomers: "P" - polysulphide; "I" - polyether, "A" - addition silicone and "Z" - condensation silicone. The angular values of the implant anangles were evaluated using a profilometer (accuracy 0.017 degrees) and then subjected to analysis of variance for comparisons at a significance level of 5% (p<0.05). For the implant analogy at 90 degrees, the "A" material associated with T2 and the "Z" material with T3 behaved differently (p<0.05) from all the groups. At 80 degrees, all the materials behaved differently (p<0.01) from T1. At 75 degrees, when T1 was associated, materials "P" and "A" showed similar behavior, as did materials "T" and "Z", however, "P" and "A" were different from "I" and "Z" (p<0.01). When T3 was associated, all the experimental groups behaved differently (p<0.01). At 65 degrees, the "P" and "Z" materials behaved differently (p<0.01) from the control group with T1, T2 and T3. The "I" and "A" materials behaved differently from the control group (p<0.01) when T1 and T2, respectively, were associated.They concluded that the more perpendicular the angle of the implant analog to the horizontal surface, the more accurate the impression. The best-performing materials, and therefore the most suitable for implant transfer impressions, were polyether and silicon adhesive, and the most satisfactory technique was the technique using square transfers bonded with acrylic resin.

Naconecy *et al.* (2004) evaluated the deformation of a metal framework connected to fifteen type IV plaster models (GC FujiRock EP) fabricated using three transfer techniques to determine the most accurate molding procedure. The impression material used was Impregum F polyether using a Pentamix®2 impression material dispenser. Three individual photoactivatable resin trays were made, two open and one closed. Five plaster models were made from impressions of an epoxy resin master model (with five implant abutment analogs) for each transfer technique. Group 1: models were created using the direct splinted technique (square transfers joined with 2.5 mm diameter carbon steel pins and GC Pattern Resin acrylic resin); Group 2: models were made using the direct unsplinted technique (square transfers); and Group 3: models were made using the indirect technique (conical transfers). Sixteen strain gauges were glued along the four surfaces of the metal structure (anterior, posterior, upper and lower) in order to capture the degree of deformation of the structure for each plaster model. The deformation data was analyzed using analysis of variance and Tukey's test at 0.05 and 0.01 levels of significance. Group 1 models allowed a more accurate reproduction of the position of the ankles compared to models made using the other techniques. No significant difference was found between the direct non-splinted technique (group 2) and the indirect technique (group 3). Although some studies have evaluated transfer techniques with similar methodology, this study demonstrated a more satisfactory distribution of strain gauges to record deformations of the structure in all directions and simultaneously compensate for the effects of temperature variation. The direct spline technique was the most accurate transfer method for multiple columns compared to the direct non-spline and indirect techniques.

Sakuno (2004) evaluated the accuracy of two impression techniques for prostheses on implants depending on the impression technique (with and without acrylic resin ferulization) and the inclination of the implant in relation to the alveolar ridge. An aluminum matrix was made into which four 3.75 mm diameter implants were inserted. The implants were inserted into the matrix so that each one had a different inclination (89.643; 74.355;59.124;45.186 degrees). These implants were molded with square transfers for internal hexagon implants (Conect Grip, Conexâo Sistemas de Prótese Ltda). Twenty casts were made, 10 of which were made without ferulization. The ferulization was done by tying the transfers with dental floss and applying acrylic resin using the brush technique. All the molds were made with a silicon adhesive. The plaster models obtained were taken to an optical microscope so that the angle formed between the surface of the plaster base and the external surface of the intermediate abutment could be measured. The results obtained, in degrees, were used to establish the distortion index for each of the molded implants. This index was calculated using the following formula: distortion index = A1 - A2, where A1 is the angle obtained for the implant in the master model and A2 is the angle measured on the corresponding implant in the plaster model. The indices were transformed into modules since the direction of the distortion was not considered relevant. The distortion index averages were calculated (for each experimental group) from 10 data points for each of the inclinations under study. The data from the experiment was treated using a two-factor analysis of variance and, when necessary, Tukey's test was used to contrast the means at an overall significance level of 5%. The factors considered in the statistical model were: a) type of impression (with and without template); and b) implant angle in the master model (89.643; 74.355; 59.124; 45.186 degrees). The results showed that the two factors under study were significant ($p < 0.05$). Thus, the overall mean distortion index when ferulization with acrylic resin was used was significantly higher (0.680 degrees) than the overall mean obtained when ferulization was not performed (0.424 degrees). The implant angle factor in the master model was also statistically significant ($p = 0.000$). The comparison between the overall averages as a function of implant angle in the master model shows that the overall average distortion index for the implant with an angle of 45.186 degrees was significantly higher than the averages for all the other angles. The interaction between the two factors studied was statistically significant ($p = 0.000$). Based on the results, it was possible to conclude that: 1) considering the Conect Grip transfer, the impression technique that does not use acrylic resin ferulization results in less distortion than the technique that uses ferulization; and 2) the inclination of the implant in relation to the alveolar ridge interferes with the distortion of the impression, with implants with less angulation (more inclined) resulting in significantly more distorted impressions.

Cabral (2005) investigated 4 printing techniques to determine their dimensional accuracy in comparison with a standard technique. A metal master framework with 2 interior hexagonal implants (SIN, Sistema de Implante Nacional Ltda. Sâo Paulo, Brazil) was used as the standard for the comparisons. Sixty master models were prepared to evaluate 4 impression techniques: (I) indirect impression technique with tapered transfer crowns; (II) indirect impression technique with non-splinted square transfer crowns; (III) direct impression technique with square transfer crowns with acrylic resin; and (IV) direct impression technique with square transfer crowns with acrylic resin splints sectioned 17 minutes after solidification and welded with the same resin. A profile projector was used to measure the distance between the crowns attached to the anangles. The average distances (mm) were calculated from 3 measurements for each sample on the master models and the master metal framework. Results: Analysis of variance and the Tukey HSD test were used for statistical analysis of the data (alpha = 0.05). The results for the direct technique with square transfer crowns with acrylic resin splints sectioned and welded after solidification were not significantly different from the results for the metal master framework. Conclusion: Considering the methodology used and the results obtained, the direct printing technique with square transfer crowns with acrylic resin splints sectioned and welded after solidification had better results than the other techniques studied.

Kim *et al.* (2006) evaluated possible displacement of implant components in a working model and suggested a method for comparing the accuracy of impression techniques during impression taking and during plaster casting. Two molding techniques were evaluated: square transfers associated with an open tray, and square transfers splinted with light-curing resin associated with an open tray. A mandibular model with five implants was made. Five working models were made per impression technique and measured using a computer that provided the coordinates of the components. The displacement data during the impression procedure and during casting were calculated. The average displacement at the moment when the protractor was attached to the replica was 31.3μm. The smallest displacement occurred in the non-splinted group compared to the splinted group during impression taking (p=.001), but when pouring the model, the non-splinted group had greater component displacement (p=.015). It can therefore be concluded that the non-splinted group was the most accurate when taking the impression, but less accurate when making the working model.

Bressani (2006) evaluated the accuracy of the implant molding procedure with a single internal hexagon using alginate and silicone adhesive. To do this, a master model was made representing a toothed mandible with an implant installed in the position of tooth 45. Five molds and five models were obtained for each material. Measurements were made with a precision caliper by three different evaluators, blind to the impression material. The analysis of variance showed no statistically significant difference between the materials evaluated. Thus, it can be concluded that the impression material did not influence the quality and accuracy of models for single implants.

Modesto (2006) compared two impression materials, a condensation silicone and a polyether, using a specific transfer molding technique. Based on a model of the human mandible with five conical abutment analogs, using the transfer molding technique with square transfers and splinted with acrylic resin and an open tray, these molding materials were compared by means of measurements taken on the models obtained. The molds were poured with special plaster, the models were photographed and the images obtained were uploaded to the imagetool image editor, where the maladjustments of the superstructure to the abutment analogues were read. He concluded that for the two impression materials, the specimens did not show statistically significant differences, however, they did show statistically significant dimensional changes in relation to the master model.

Rodrigues (2006) evaluated 2 transfer molding techniques used in prostheses on implants, varying the joining methods between the transfers. From a metal base containing 3 implant analogs, a metal bar was placed using the laser welding method. Twenty individual impression trays were then made from self-curing acrylic resin to take 5 impressions for each group, divided as follows: Group A - square transfers bonded with dental floss and covered with acrylic resin (Duralay); Group B - square transfers bonded with prefabricated acrylic resin bars (Duralay); Group C - conical transfers (without bonding); Group D - square transfers bonded with light-curing acrylic resin. The molding material chosen for all groups was Impregum polyether and Fuji Rock plaster. For measurement, the bar was screwed from left to right into each of the 20 specimens obtained and the dimensional change values were read using an optical microscope at 100X magnification. To do this, a comparison was made with the metal base, measuring the areas formed between the analogues present in the models and the metal bar. According to the results, there was no statistically significant difference between the techniques and the groups, although Group B, which used prefabricated bars made of self-curing acrylic resin, showed a misfit closer to that of the laser-welded bar.

Chavez (2007) evaluated, *in vitro,* the accuracy of a registration technique (Index) and three molding techniques (Square transfers, Joined squares and Squares with helix-shaped extensions) associated with two clinical situations (aligned and non-aligned ananglasts). All the prosthetic components used were made by Conexâo (Conexâo Sistemas de Prótese). An epoxy resin master model was built, simulating a partially edentulous lower arch, on which six Micro-Unit abutment rings were fixed. Two three-element metal frameworks, three aligned and three non-aligned, and twenty-one individual acrylic resin impression trays were made. The molding material used was polyether (Impregum Soft Medium Viscosity - 3M ESPE) and the plaster used was type IV plaster (FujiRock -GC Corp), vacuum sprayed. A total of twenty-one models were obtained, seven per technique, plus seven index records. These measurements were made using a program (Leica QWin) which received the images from a video camera coupled to a Leica magnifying glass (100x magnification). The gaps obtained were: Master model = 32.28µm; Index = 34.26µm; Square = 75.80µm; Joined square = 56.00µm; Helix square = 39.80µm; and for the arrangement of the implants the gaps were: Aligned = 50.940µm and Non-aligned = 65.357µm. The statistical tests used were Student Newman-Keuls and Kruskal-Wallis ($\square$=0.05). It was concluded that in relation to the techniques studied: 1- The most accurate technique was the index; 2- The best molding technique was the one with square transfers with helix; 3 The clinical situation that promoted the most accurate model was the one with aligned anangles.

Conrad (2007) analyzed the effect of the combined interaction of the impression technique for angled implants and the number of implants on the accuracy of definitive models. A definitive stone model was fabricated for each of the 6 experimental groups and 1 control group. All 7 definitive models had 3 implants arranged in a triangular test pattern creating a plane. In the 6 experimental groups, the central implant was perpendicular to the plane of the model when the outer implants had 5, 10, or 15 degrees of convergence to or divergence from the central implant. The definitive control model had all 3 implants parallel to each other and perpendicular to the plane of the model. Five open trays and 5 closed trays were used together with silicone adhesive to obtain each definitive model. The impressions were cast with type IV stone, and a fine-tipped measuring stylus was used to record multiple centerline coordinates (X-Y-Z) on the upper surface of the implant hexagon and at the base of the model. Computer software was used to align the data series and the vector calculations determined the difference in degrees between the implant angles in the definitive model and the duplicate models. Statistical analysis for repeated measures ANOVA (α=.05). It concluded that the angle errors for the open tray techniques did not differ significantly (P=.22). The angulation of the implants and the number of implants differed in the mean angle errors but not in the entire easily interpreted standard test (P<.001). The combined interaction of impression technique, implant angulation, and number of implants had no effect on the accuracy of duplicate models compared to definitive models (P=.19). The mean angle errors for impressions with open trays did not differ significantly. There was no interpretable standard test of the mean angle errors in terms of implant angulation and the number of implants. The distortion value was similar for all combinations of impression technique, implant angulation and number of implants.

Del'Acqua *et al.* (2008) evaluated the accuracy of a registration technique (Index) and three molding techniques (conical, square and joined square transfers) associated with three pouring techniques (Conventional, with Latex tubes and with an analogue joined with Duralay) for implant-supported prostheses. All the prosthetic components used came from Conexâo (Conexâo Sistemas de Prótese). A brass master model was built simulating an edentulous lower arch, where four Micro-Unit abutment rings were provisionally fixed perpendicular to the surface and parallel to each other, called rings A, B, C and D. A metal structure was fabricated and screwed to the four new abutments. This set was passively cemented to the master model with epoxy resin. An individual aluminum tray was made (with 2mm of relief) for the technique with the joined square transfers and another for the techniques with the conical and square transfers. The molding material used was polyether (Impregum Soft Medium Viscosity - 3M ESPE) and the plaster used was a type IV plaster (Vel-Mix, Kerr), vacuum-sprayed. A load of 1250g was placed on the tray to standardize the pressure during impression taking. A total of fifty models were obtained, five per technique. The metal structure was screwed in place with a torque of 10 Ncm on all models in an analog A, while measurements of the cracks formed were made in an anogs C and D. This process was repeated in an analog D, noting the measurements from anogs A and B. These measurements were made using a program (Leica QWin) that received the images from a video camera coupled to a Leica magnifying glass (100x magnification). The slits obtained were: Master model = 31.63 µm; Index = 27.07 µm; Conical / Conventional = 116.97 µm; Conical / Làtex = 65.69 µm; Conical / Duralay = 141.12 µm; Square / Conventional = 57.84 µm; Square / Làtex = 38.03 µm; Square / Duralay = 74.19 µm; Joined square / Conventional = 73.17 µm; Joined square / Làtex = 82.47 µm; Joined square / Duralay = 104.67 µm. The statistical tests used were Mann-Whitney, Kruskal-Wallis, Tukey and Dunn (a=0.05). It can be concluded that in relation to the techniques studied: 1- The best molding technique was the one with square transfers; 2- The best pouring technique, whether molding with conical or square transfers, was the technique that used latex tubes; 3- The form of pouring did not influence the accuracy of the plaster models for the technique with the joined square transfers; 4- The Index or Square / Latex techniques accurately transfer the positioning of the implants, being statistically similar to the master model.

Lopes Junior (2008) evaluated the dimensional stability of three direct implant position transfer techniques and four RAAQ (Duralay I, Duralay II, GC Pattern and Dencrilay), over four different periods, using the photoelasticity technique. Three photoelastic models were made containing two 13mm long implants with a 4.1mm platform. Two square transfers were screwed onto these and splinted with RAAQ in three different ways: with metal rods, prefabricated acrylic bars and with dental floss. Photoelastic analysis was carried out using a circular polariscope at four different times (20 minutes, 3, 24 and 36 hours) and made it possible to calculate the distortion energy (E) in the apical region of the implants and the force generated on the transfers in each experiment. The results were statistically analyzed (p<0.05) and, when comparing the four resins, there was a statistically significant difference when the prefabricated bar technique (p=0.000) and dental floss (p=0.001) were used. However, when the metal rod technique was used, no significant difference was found (p=0.116). Dencrilay resin showed greater dimensional changes, both in the bar and floss techniques. Duralay II and GC showed the lowest values when applied to the prefabricated bar and Duralay I and GC showed the lowest values for dental floss. When comparing the techniques, the one with metal rods showed the lowest values for Duralay I, GC and Dencrilay resins. For the prefabricated bar technique, the Duralay II resin generated the lowest values. For all resins, the flossing technique showed the worst results. The transfer technique with metal rods was the most appropriate and the resins with the lowest dimensional changes were Duralay I, Duralay II and GC Pattern.

Ribas (2008) compared five different direct molding techniques (n=5): group 1- separate transfers, group 2- transfers bonded with acrylic resin, group 3- transfers bonded with acrylic resin, segmented and bonded again with acrylic resin, group 4- transfers coated with the adhesive of the molding material and group 5- transfers bonded with acrylic resin, separated and bonded again with cyanoacrylate and with a latex tube over the analogue in order to provide a double casting of plaster. To do this, an acrylic resin matrix was made in which four 4.1 mm external hexagon implants were fixed. The implants were molded using individualized trays made of acrylic and polyether. A total of 25 models with 100 measurements were taken. All measurements were made using a comparative microscope. The average mismatches measured were: 6.42µm for group 1, 11.53µm in group 2, in group 3 it was 7.03µm and in groups 4 and 5, 5.12 and 6.10µm, respectively. There was no statistically significant difference between the groups with bonded and unbonded transfers. The worst results were shown by group 2.

Lee *et al.* (2008) carried out a systematic review to investigate the accuracy of published transfer impression techniques for implants, and also to examine the clinical factors that could affect the accuracy of these impressions. The electronic search was carried out in June 2008 in MEDLINE, EMBASE and Cochrane Library databases with the keywords, implants, impression and impressions. The study investigated the accuracy of implant impressions in articles published in English. In addition, a manual search was carried out to enrich the results in the time period from January 1980 to May 2008. After carrying out the search strategies, 41 articles were selected for inclusion in the review process. Results: All the articles selected were *in vitro* studies. Of the 17 studies that compared the accuracy of the splinted and unsplinted techniques, 7 advocated the splinted technique, 3 advocated the unsplinted technique and 7 reported no difference. Fourteen studies compared the accuracy of transfer techniques The number of implants is important when comparing splinted and unsplinted techniques. Eleven studies compared the accuracy of polyether and vinyl polysiloxane materials and 10 reported no difference between the two. Four studies examined the effect of implant angulation on the accuracy of impression techniques. Two studies reported high accuracy with straight implants, while another two reported that implant angulation had no effect. Conclusion: In the review regarding the level of the implant connection, the splinted technique is more accurate. For situations in which there were 3 or fewer implants, most studies showed no difference between the techniques, whereas for 4 or more implants, most studies showed more accuracy with the splinted transfer technique. Polyether and VPS are the most suitable materials for implant transfer impressions.

Augustin *et al.* (2009) evaluated the polymerization contraction of Luxatemp Sterngold resin (DMG-Hamburg-Germany) in the bonding of impression transfers for prostheses on implants. An acrylic model with 4 implants was built on a semi-adjustable articulator (ASA) plate. Mini abutments were installed on these. The model was taken to the Ericson platform and measured in millimeters at the upper end of the abutments. Transfers were then installed and measurements were taken on the upper base of the transfer and the screw. These were taken by 3 examiners. The transfers were bonded in two ways: Group 01: Pattern; Group 02: Sterngold. After polymerization, the set was removed, an analog installed and plaster inserted into an ASA plate. Ten models were made for each group. The same measurements were taken on the plaster model. Distortion was assessed using the distance between the abutments and transfers in the initial and final models. The result for group 01 was 0.12983mm and for group 02 0.15700mm. There was no statistical difference (Mann-Whitney). This methodology led to the conclusion that Sterngold resin did not show significantly different polymerization contraction from Pattern resin and can be used in the transfer ferulization of implant dentistry impressions.

Alves Junior *et al.* (2009) evaluated and compared 3 transfer molding techniques for implants, using 3 different molding materials and stock trays. The null hypothesis is that the use of acrylic resin to splint the copings may be able to prevent the displacement of the transfers within the impression by preventing micro-movements. A master model was made to simulate a clinical situation where the location of multiple implants had to be recorded. Thirty impressions were made using 3 techniques: silicone adhesive (control); acrylic resin and condensation silicone (test 1); and irreversible hydrocolloid and acrylic resin (test 2). A profile projector was used to measure the distance between the implant rings in the models produced and the data were recorded for statistical analysis. The groups had a normal distribution (Shapiro-Wilk, p>0.05) and no statistically significant differences (ANOVA, p>0.05). They concluded that splinted transfers are less susceptible to small movements within the impression material, producing more homogeneous results.

Gennari Filho *et al.* (2009) compared splinting techniques for transfer molding of osseointegrated implants with different angulations. A metal matrix containing two replicas of implants (control) at 90 degrees and 65 degrees to the horizontal plane was used for the four impression techniques: Technique 1 (T1), direct technique, square transfers without joining in an open tray; Technique 2   (T2), square transfers,

Technique 3 (T3), square transfers, splinted with dental floss and self-curing acrylic resin; Technique 4 (T4), square transfers, splinted with prefabricated resin bars. The impression material used was polyether. The replicas were scanned to capture the images which were evaluated individually in a computer graphics program. The program made it possible to read the angle between the replicas and the base. The images of the replicas were compared with the image of the matrix (control) and the differences in angulation of the image of the control group were calculated. Analysis of variance and Tukey's test were used for statistical analysis (p<0.05). Results: All groups showed significant differences in implant angulations compared to the control group (p<0.05). Group T1 showed the highest difference (1.019 degrees) followed by groups T2 (0.747 degrees), T3 (0.516 degrees), and T4 (0.325 degrees) which showed the lowest angular change compared to the control group. There were significant differences between tilted and right-angled implants in all groups except group T4. Conclusion: Based on the results obtained, the following conclusions can be drawn: All the replicas obtained with the transfer molds showed different angulations in relation to the matrix; the implants with an angulation of 65 degrees showed the highest differences in angulation when compared to the matrix; the T1 technique (direct without joining in an open tray) showed the greatest difference when compared to the matrix; the T4 technique (splinted with prefabricated resin bars) showed the best result among the techniques evaluated.

3. Proposition

The purpose of this study was to evaluate four transfer molding techniques for osseointegrated implants with regard to marginal misalignments and stresses induced in the metallic superstructure:

-   moldings with conical transfers;

-   moldings with unjointed square transfers;

-   moldings with square transfers joined with chemically activated acrylic resin rods;

-   moldings with square transfers bonded with self-curing bis-acrylic composite resin.

4. Materials and Methods

General Design

A metal matrix was made in which three replicas of 3.75 mm external hexagon implants (Conexao Sistemas de Prótese Ltda; Sao Paulo-SP) were fixed to simulate a clinical situation.

Characteristics of the metal matrix.

The metal matrix used in this study was made from a stainless steel *chassis* (Kleine, 2002; Daroz, 2006; Spazzin, 2009), on which three replicas of osseointegrated implants with a 3.75 mm cervical platform and an external hexagonal prosthetic connection (Connection) were placed, arranged to represent a clinical situation in the lower arch. The replicas were positioned using a Delineator (BioArt-Sao Carlos-SP) and fixed to the matrix *chassis* using transverse screws (Figure 1).

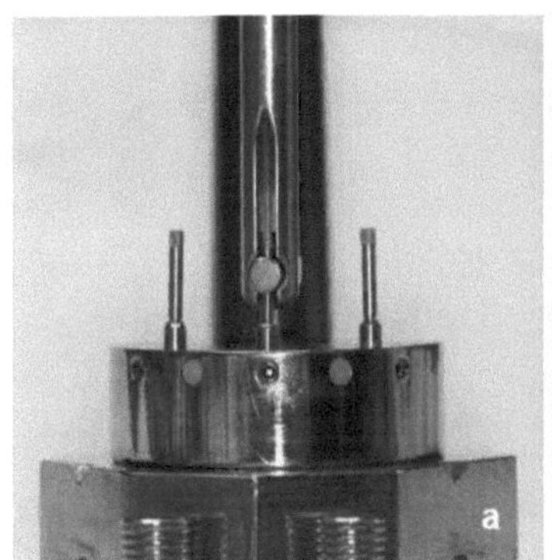
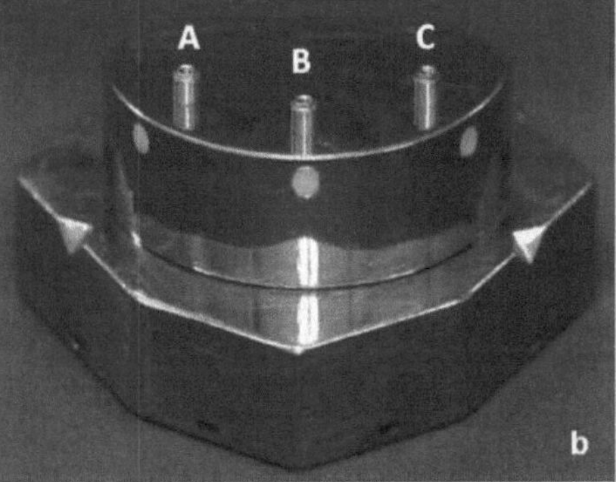

Figure 1. a) Replicas being positioned in the metal matrix; b) metal matrix with the replicas positioned.

Metal superstructure

To obtain the superstructure, intermediate UCLA-type pillars for multiple parts (Conexao) were fitted directly onto the replicas and fixed in place using corresponding screws. The superstructure, which was made to a specific size and configuration to allow the attachment of strain gauges for stress capture and strain gauge evaluation, was waxed, included and cast in a cobalt chromium alloy, Star Loy C (DeguDent GmbH-Rodenbacher Chaussee 463457 Hanau - Wolfgang- Germany) (Figure 2).

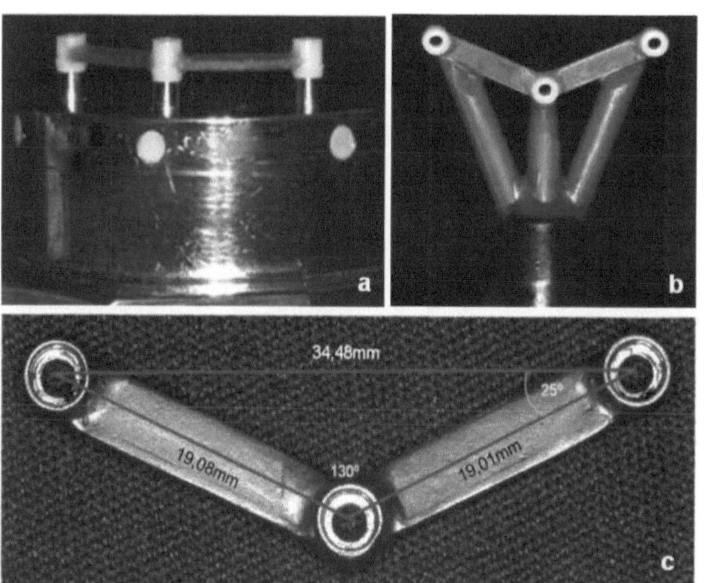

Figure 2. a) Structure waxed on the matrix b) on the base for casting; c) after finishing, with the specific measurements.

Individual molds

Individual molds were made to carry out the procedures.

After positioning the transfers on the ananglasts, the matrix, ananglasts and transfers were waxed up, relieved with a 1.5 mm thick sheet of pink wax No. 7 (Wilson-Labordental SP), plus a 0.5 mm thick sheet of Roach casting wax (Wilson-Labordental-SP), providing a 2 mm relief for the impression material.

The waxed set was then molded with an individualized stock tray and Alginate (Jeltrate - Dentsply-RJ). The mold was poured with special type IV plaster (Resin Rock-Whip Mix-USA), thus obtaining a model with the dimensions of the master model relieved in wax, on which the individual tray was waxed up with a thickness of 3mm and its own individual characteristics (Figure 3. a and b).

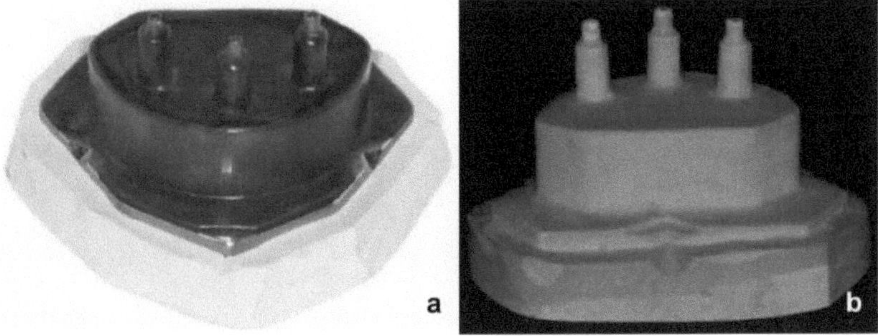

Figure 3. a) Wax relief; b) plaster model for making the trays.

Because the resulting volume of the waxed tray was very large, it was necessary to make an individual muffle out of special plaster so that the individual trays could be polymerized (Figure 4. a, b and c).

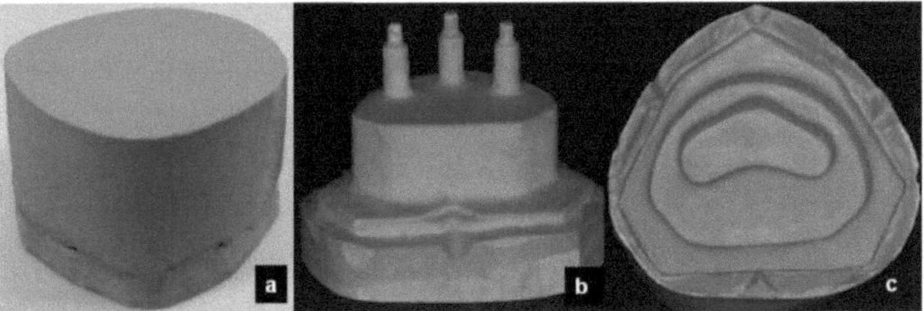

Figure 4. a) Plaster muffle; b) plaster model for making the trays; c) plaster muffle, internal view.

All four individual trays (one for each technique) were made from chemically activated acrylic resin (Artigos Odontológico Clàssico Ltda. - Sâo Paulo - SP). After finishing, the handle and two supports at the back were attached to provide support when taking impressions and pouring the plaster.

Matrix for molding and pouring the plaster

A matrix for molding and pouring the plaster was made from addition-curing silicone (Reprosil - Dentsply - USA). This matrix was used for all the impressions and filling of the plaster mould, allowing the moulds and the shape of the plaster models to be standardized, as well as the amount of plaster used for filling (Del'Acqua *et al.*, 2008) (Figure 5).

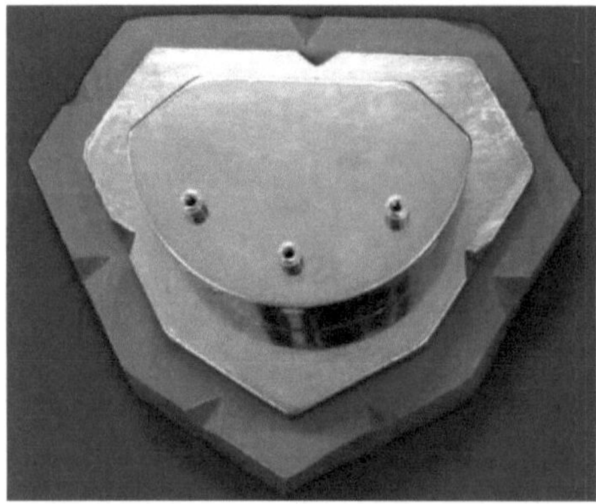

Figure 5: Silicone matrix in position.

<u>*The techniques studied were:*</u>

Conical transfers

The conical transfers were manually screwed into the master model's anangles until some resistance was felt and then with the help of the internal friction wrench (Figure 6).

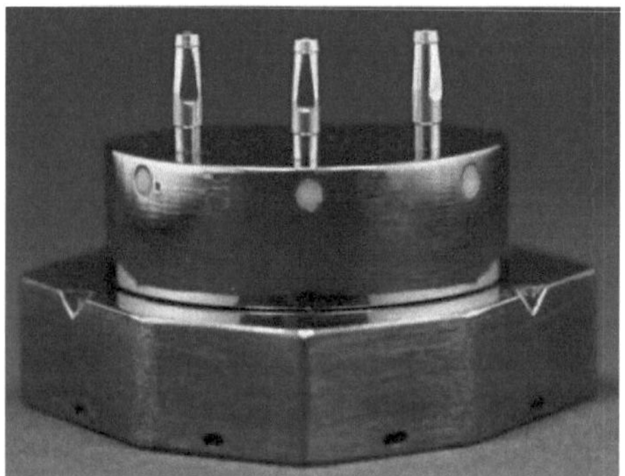

Figure 6 - Conical transfers attached to the metal matrix.

Insulated square transfers

The square transfers were screwed in using a 1.17 mm external hexagon hand wrench until resistance was felt and then torqued to 20 Ncm using a calibrated prosthetic torque wrench (Conexao) (Ivanhoe *et al.*, 1991). The sequence of screw tightening was always from the central abutment to one of the ends. All screws were retorqued 10 minutes after the initial torque of 20 Ncm (Jemt, 1991 and Siamos *et al.*, 2002).

Square transfers joined with prefabricated resin rods.

All the transfers were placed on the replicas, initially by hand tightening and then using a prosthetic torque wrench (Conexao) with a torque of 20 Ncm. We waited 10 minutes and retorqued.

The transfers were joined by applying Pattern acrylic resin around the retaining part of the square transfers.

Bars of chemically activated acrylic resin were made by injecting the resin into plastic straws with a diameter of 3 mm (Quick Ind. e Com. Ltda - Limeira-SP), using a hypodermic plastic syringe. After 20 minutes, the resin bar was removed from the straw, the diameter was checked with a caliper and it was stored in water to be used only after 24 hours (Del'Acqua et al., 2008).

The resin bars were sectioned into appropriate lengths to close the gap between adjacent transfers. The ends of the resin bars were bonded to the transfers using the Nealon technique, in which a quantity of polymer is captured using a brush soaked in monomer (Figure 7).

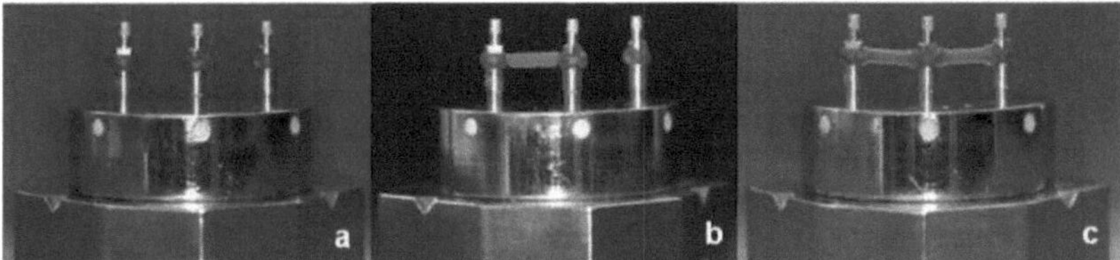

Figure 7. a) Square transfers with resin around the retentive area; b) resin rod cut out in position to be fixed; c) resin rods fixed.

To minimize the changes that occur during the polymerization of the resin, sections were made in the middle of the bars and the transfers were tightened again with a torque of 20 Ncm.

After cutting, the bars were joined again with Pattern acrylic resin using the Nealon technique, waiting 20 minutes before molding (Del'Acqua *et al.,* 2008) (Figure 8).

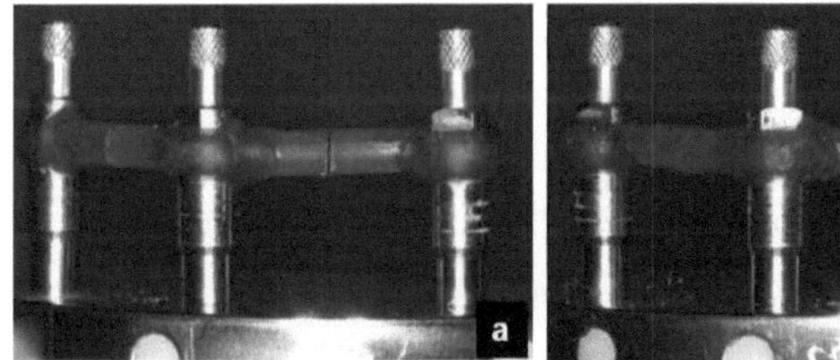

Figure 8. a) Resin rod sectioned; b) rods rejoined with resin.

The same acrylic resin splinting described above was used to transfer the molding components to all ten models made with the splinted technique, but the splint was sectioned and re-bonded as described above before each impression (Burawi *et al.*, 1997; and Del'Acqua *et al.*, 2008).

Square transfers bonded with bis-acrylic resin

Characteristics of *bis-acrylic* resin (DMG Chemisch- Pharmazeutische Hamburg - Germany) according to the manufacturer: It is a self-hardening composite for making crowns and temporary fixed prostheses, inlays, onlays and veneers. The material consists of 2 components based on multifunctional methacrylates. It is mixed in the cannula by actuating the lever on the output device and can be applied directly.

Form of presentation - Starter pack: 1 cartridge with 76g of paste in A2 color, 15 automix-Tips, 1 automix Dispenser.

Composition - Vitreous filler in a matrix of multifunctional methacrylates, catalysts, stabilizers and additives, free of methylmethacrylate and peroxides.

Percentage of filling material - 44% by weight =24% by volume.

Technical Data

Pressure resistance   250 MPa

Flexural strength   91.5 MPa

Diametral tensile strength36   MPa

Hardness Barcol37

Water absorption   0.76% by weight

Maximum hardening temperature   ≈ 38°C

Polymerization shrinkage7   .6 - 8%

Working time management: 0 - 45 sec - Insertion into mouth

6 - 7 min - Mouth removal

The transfers were joined by placing a piece of tension-free dental floss around the retaining part of the square transfers.

Next, the resin was applied evenly over the floss tie to make a bar with a diameter of approximately 3mm (Figures 9 and 10).

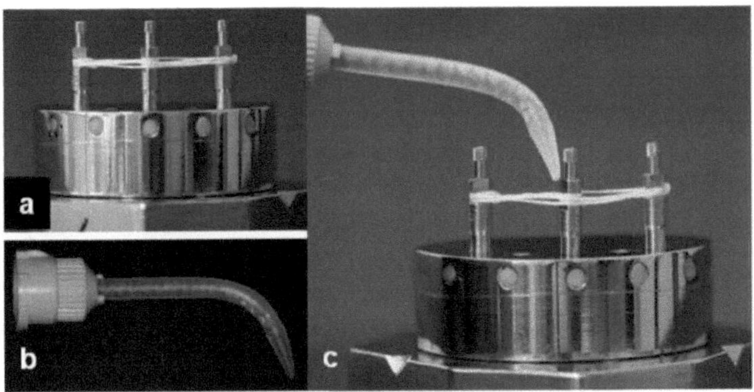

Figure 9. a) Transfers with floss ties; b) modified self-mixing applicator tip; c) tip in position to apply the resin over the tie.

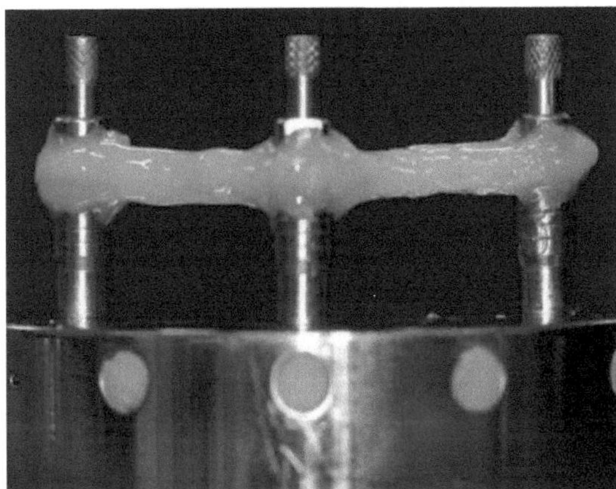

Figure 10. Splinting completed.

Molding procedures

All procedures were carried out at an ambient temperature of (23°C ± 2°C) and relative humidity of 66% ± 10%. Ten impressions were taken for each technique.

The seating surfaces of all components were cleaned with isopropyl alcohol before each procedure (Burawi *et al.,* 1997 and Del'Acqua *et al.,* 2008).

The fit of the transfers to the analogues was checked visually under strong lighting and with the aid of a lapel magnifier with four times magnification (BioArt -Sâo Carlos - Sâo Paulo), during all the molding and filling procedures.

Before each new impression, all the impression material and adhesive were removed (Thinner Luksnova.206-SP-Brazil) and the tray was degreased with isopropyl alcohol. A new layer of adhesive was then applied.

The molding material used for all techniques was Honigum-Mono single-component silicone (DMG Chemisch-Pharmazeutische Hamburg-Germany).

Molding

The individual acrylic resin trays, one for each technique, were previously treated with a thin layer of tray adhesive (3M ESPE-Germany) applied with a brush to the entire inner surface and 3 mm beyond the edges (Figure 11).

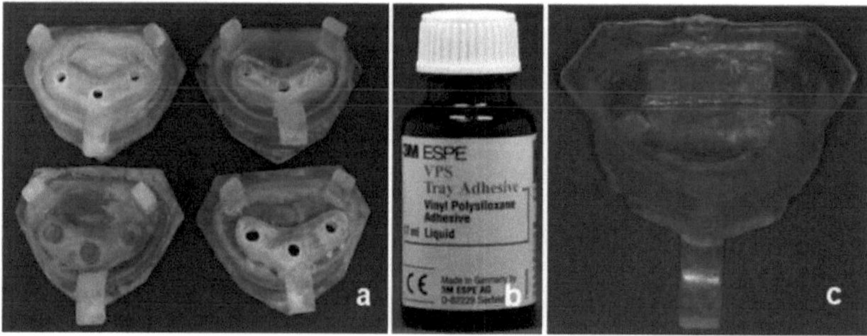

Figure 11 (a) Individual trays; (b) Adhesive for tray; (c) Tray after application of adhesive.

The order of the molding procedures, according to the groups, was chosen by lot.

After applying the adhesive, we waited 15 minutes. The impression material was prepared and placed in the dispenser according to the manufacturer's recommendations.

The impression material was then first placed in the tray, then injected around the transfers. Next, the tray (which had fittings so that it could always be placed in the same position on the model) was seated by applying bidigital pressure until the fittings contacted the base of the master model, remaining in this position for 10 minutes.

In order to standardize the pressure during molding, a load of 1250g was placed on the tray to keep it in position, leaving the molding material confined under constant pressure (Del'Acqua *et al.*, 2008) (Figure 12).

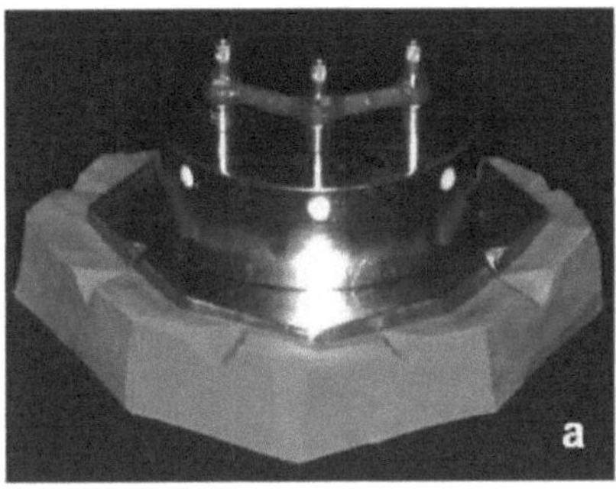
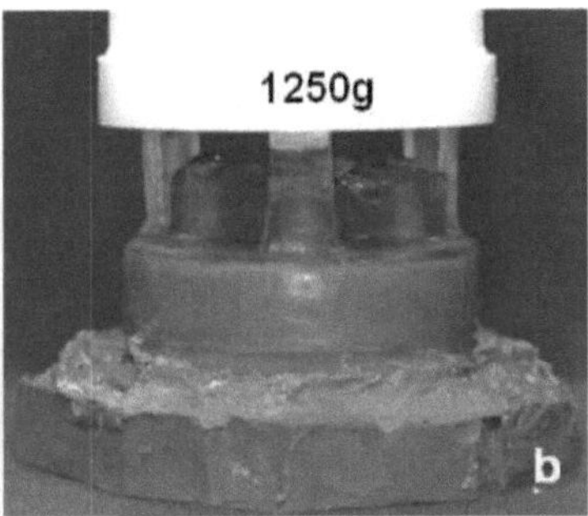

Figure 12. a) Matrix for filling the mold with plaster, in position; b) mold in position, with the specific load to maintain constant molding pressure.

Once the stipulated setting time of 10 minutes had elapsed, the load placed on the tray was removed and the mold was separated from the matrix. After 30 minutes, the mold/matrix was separated so that the silicone could recover the deformations it had undergone during the separation procedure, the analogues were positioned, followed by the latex tubes and the mold was filled with plaster.

For all the procedures, the special low expansion resin plaster, Resin Rock (Whip Mix - USA), was used, proportioned according to the manufacturer's recommendations, i.e. 20ml of water for 100g of powder, mixed with distilled water, initially manually for 15 seconds and then mechanically spatulated for a further 30 seconds in the Degussa vacuum spatulator (Degussa Sâo Paulo, SP).

Each mold was first filled using the Latex tube technique (McCartney & Pearson, 1994; Del'Acqua *et al., 2008),* 2008) involving the analogs, after the initial setting of the plaster (30 minutes), the latex tubes were removed, the plaster was hydrated for 5 minutes, the matrix for filling the plaster was positioned in the mold, a new portion of plaster was prepared and poured, first in the spaces left by the latex tubes under constant vibration provided by the plaster vibrator of the spatulator itself, aided by a dripper, continuing until the mold was completely filled, according to the conventional technique (Figures 13 and 14).

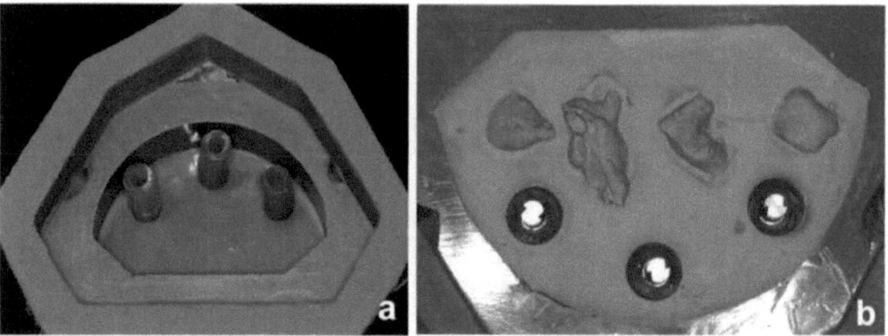

Figure 13. a) Mold with the latex tubes in place; b) 30 minutes later, with the latex tubes removed.

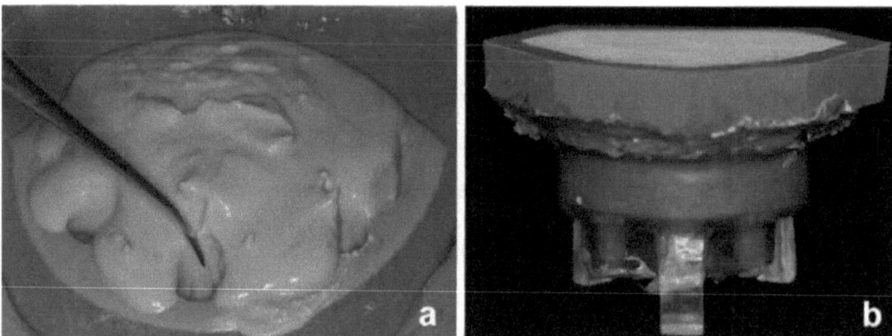

Figure 14. a) Filling the second portion of plaster with the aid of the dripper; b) set, mold/mould in position awaiting the final setting time of the plaster.

Only one plaster cast was made in each mold. The model had to be separated from the mold within one hour of the last filling.

The base and sides of the plaster models were smoothed with 400-grit sandpaper for a better finish.

For the square transfer technique, after the plaster had set, the screws were unscrewed and then the mold/model set was separated.

For the technique using conical transfers, the mold/model set was first separated and then the conical transfers on the plaster model were unscrewed.

After all the models had been made, i.e. 10 for each technique, they were stored at room temperature for a week until the measurements were taken.

Measuring marginal mismatches

Marginal misalignments were measured according to the following protocol:

The metal superstructure and the replicas were first cleaned with isopropyl alcohol. The structure was then placed on the replicas positioned on the model, the fixing screws were placed in position and screwed in gently by hand, starting with the central pillar until the structure was seated on the replica. This procedure was carried out for all three pillars. Next, using a prosthetic torque wrench, a torque of 20Ncm was applied, in accordance with the manufacturer's recommendations. We waited 10 minutes and retorqued, then began the reading procedures. The first screw to be tightened was always the central one and then one of the A or C loops, also determined by lot.

Before starting the torque procedures, the prosthetic torque wrench was calibrated with a digital torque wrench.

Misalignment was defined as the vertical distance in micrometres (µm) from the edge of the metal structure to the edge of the abutment.

The order of the measurements was determined by drawing lots among the pillars. The misalignments were measured by direct visualization at 120x magnification using a measuring microscope with a precision of 1.0 µm (UHL VMM-100-BT; United Kingdom), equipped with a digital camera (KC-512NT; Kodo BR Eletrônica Ltda; Sâo Paulo, SP) and an analyzer unit (QC 220-HH Quadra-Check 200; Metronics Inc., Bedford, United States) (Figures 15 and 16).

The readings of the misalignments in the models were also determined by lot, both for the types of moldings and for the order of the abutments to be measured.

Marginal misalignments in the models were measured according to the following protocol:

The structure was placed on the replicas located on the model, the fixing screws were placed in position and screwed in gently by hand, starting with the central pillar until the structure was seated on the replica. This procedure was carried out for all three pillars. Next, using a prosthetic torque wrench, a torque of 20Ncm was applied, in accordance with the manufacturer's recommendations. We waited 10 minutes and retorqued the abutments, before starting the reading procedures. The first screw to be tightened was always the central abutment (B), followed by A or C, also determined by lot.

The misfit readings were taken at the structure/replicas interface, at points marked on the buccal and lingual faces of each abutment and were repeated consecutively three times, the average of these repetitions being considered the average marginal misfit (Figure 16).

After each sequence of readings, a new set of prosthetic screws was used.

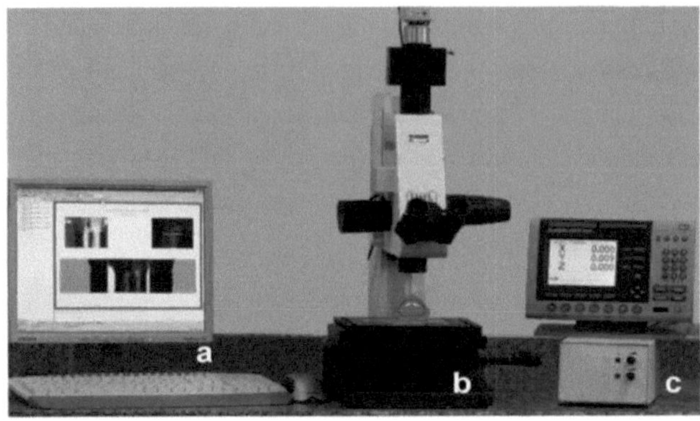

Figure 15. Reading instruments: (a) Monitor; (b) Microscope; (c) Checkerboard.

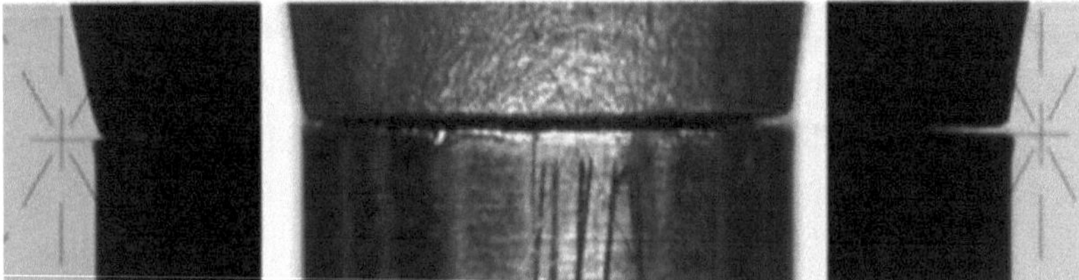

Figure 16. Visualization of the misfit by transillumination at 120 X magnification.

Voltage measurement

The stresses were measured using two electrical resistance strain *gauges* (PA-06-060BG-350L, Excel Engenharia de Sensores; Embu, São Paulo) - positioned directly on the superstructure, top and bottom (Figures 17, 19 and 20). The arrangement of the strain gauges in each fixture, i.e. each pair of strain gauges, located on diametrically opposite surfaces to each other, formed a ½ Wheatstone bridge connection responsible for a deformation reading channel.

Electrical resistance extensometers, also called transducers, are elements that transform small variations in dimensions into equivalent variations in electrical resistance. When glued to the surface of a given material, they follow the deformation to which this material is subjected, changing the resistance to the passage of the low-intensity electric current that runs through them. Their use provides a means of measuring and recording the phenomenon of deformation as an electrical quantity (Figure 17).

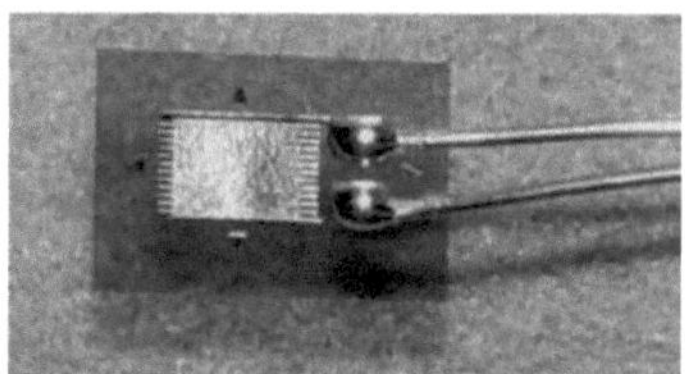

Figure 17. Electrical resistance extensometer.

The tension was calculated by reading the elastic deformations suffered by the loops. To make sure that the superstructure had not suffered plastic deformations, after reading each loop, the tension values were checked to see if they returned to zero. In order for the strain gauges to detect the micro-deformations of a surface, it was necessary for there to be intimate and effective contact between the two. To do this, the surface of the metal structure was not only polished, but also cleaned with isopropyl alcohol to remove any grease. A small amount of adhesive (Loctite 406, Henkel Loctite Adesivos Ltda., Itapevi-Sâo Paulo) was applied to the contact surface of the strain gauges which, once properly positioned, were subjected to digital pressure interposed by a soft plastic sheet for a period of 3 minutes.

The electrical signals were captured by a computer-controlled device (ASD0500; Lynx Tecnologia Eletrônica Ltda, Sâo Paulo, SP) and processed by specific *software* (AqDados 7; Lynx) (Koke *et al.*, 2004; Naconecy et *al.*, 2004; Tramontino *et al.*, 2008; Daroz, 2009) (Figure 18).

The following protocol was followed: The anangluses were given the names A, B and C, the superstructure was positioned over the replicas on the model, seated, the screws were placed in position and tightened manually with the aid of a digital key, always starting with the central ananglogue followed by the two adjacent to it (Jemt, 1991), ending with the aid of a torque wrench (Conexâo Sistemas de Prótese - Sâo Paulo - SP) and a torque of 20 Ncm on the corresponding prosthetic screws (Watanabe *et al.*, 2000.

Before starting the readings, the device was calibrated according to the manufacturer's recommendations.

The 40 models were distributed and analyzed in sequence by drawing lots. The readings were taken by the same operator and always in triplicate, from which the average was taken. After each sequence of readings, a new set of prosthetic screws was used.

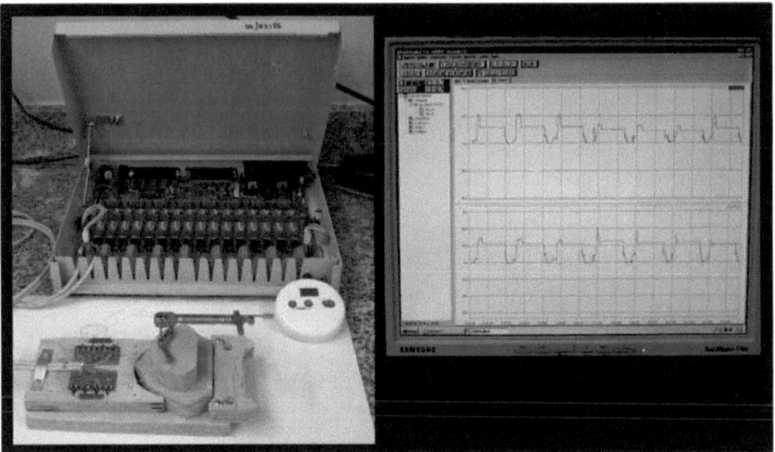

Figura 18. Voltage reading equipment; reading being carried out on one of the models.

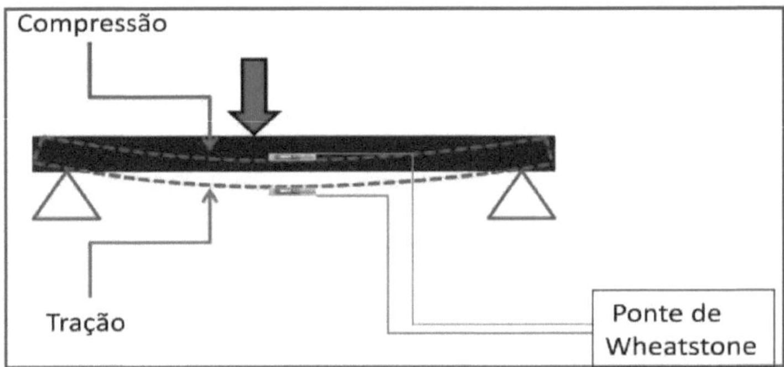

Figura 19. Schematic drawing of the extensometric reading of a structure under deformation (bending).

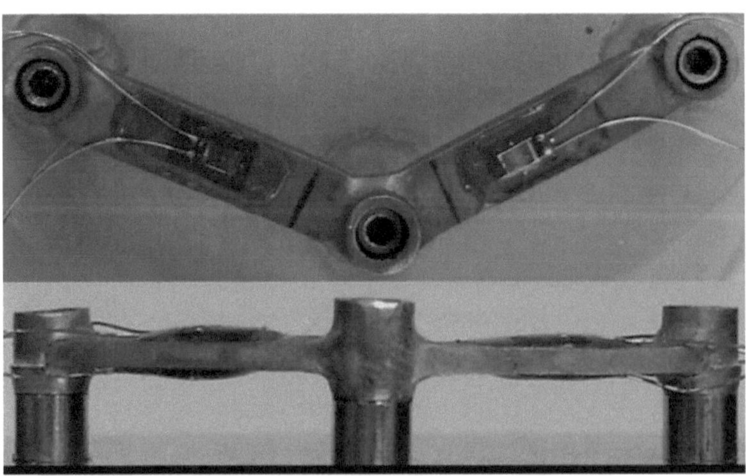

Figure 20. Extensometers attached to the superstructure.

Statistical analysis

The Kruskal-Wallis non-parametric test was used to compare the groups, with a significance level of 5%.

The Pearson correlation coefficient formula was used to calculate the correlation coefficient, followed by a hypothesis test to check whether the value of the coefficient found can be accepted as significant. Again, the significance level adopted was 5%. The database was built using Excel software and the statistical tests were carried out using the BioEstat 4.0 program.

Four groups were analyzed, each group having ten repetitions (models). The analysis variables were **tension** and **misfit**.

The Shapiro-Wilk test was used to verify the normality of the data at a significance level of 5%. For the misfit variable the test value was W=0.3512 with p-value = 0.0001 and for the tension variable the test value was W=0.7875 with p-value = 0.0001. Since both p-values were lower than the set level (5%), it is not possible to admit the normality of the data. Therefore, the Kruskal-Wallis non-parametric statistical test was used to verify the existence of a significant difference between the groups with regard to the two variables studied. Multiple comparisons, also non-parametric, were used to indicate which group or groups led to statistical significance.

5. Results

Using the Kruskal-Wallis test for multiple comparisons, it was found that for the **tension** variable the p-value was p= 0.0043 and for the **misfit** variable the p-value was p= 0.6073. Since α was set at 0.05, it was possible to infer that only for the tension variable did the groups show statistically significant differences.

Table 1 and figure 21 show the means (standard deviation) of the **tension** values according to the experimental groups. The results indicate that the lowest average tension was observed with Group C, when compared to the other groups, which did not differ significantly from each other.

Table 1. Average tension values (gf) (standard deviation) according to the experimental groups.

Group	Tension gf (dp)
Group A	8359,15 (2287,82) a
Group B	10037,63 (4953,50) a
Group C	5859,66 (976,14) b
Group D	7590,84(1782,14) a

Averages followed by different letters differed according to the Kruskal-Wallis test (α=0.05).

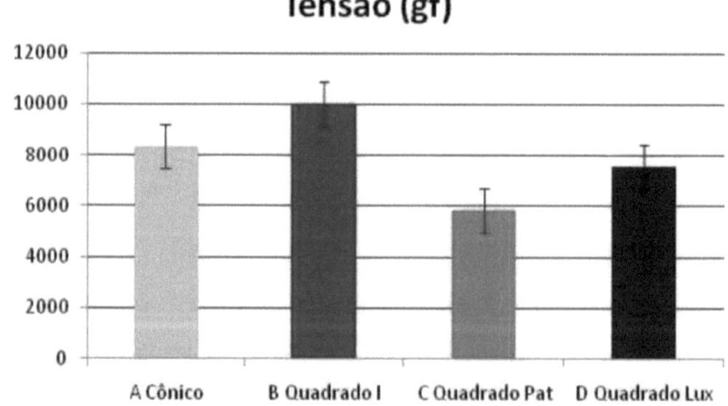

Figure 21. Graph of the mean stress values (gf) according to the experimental groups.

Table 2 and figure 22 show the means (standard deviation) of the **marginal misfit** values (μm) according to the experimental groups. The Kruskal-Wallis test showed no significant difference between the groups.

Table 2. Average marginal misfit values (μm) according to the experimental groups.

Group	Marginal misalignment μm (dp)
Group A	16 (0,005) a
Group B	26 (0,031) a
Group C	14 (0,002) a
Group D	15 (0,003) a

Averages followed by different letters differed according to the Kruskal-Wallis test (α=0.05).

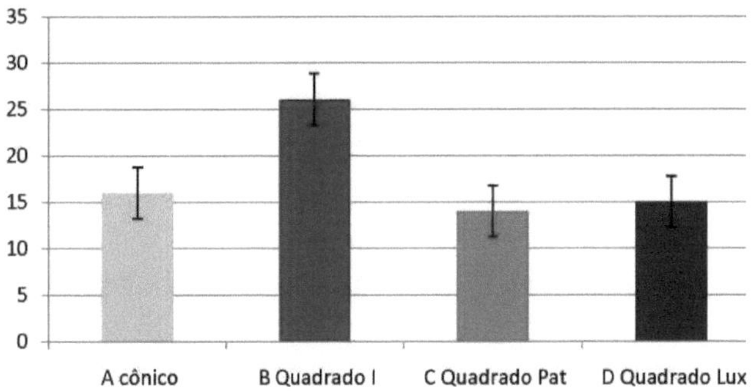

Figura 22   Graph of the mean marginal misfit values (μm) according to the experimental groups.

Correlation Coefficient

The possible correlation between marginal misfit and tension values was analyzed. To do this, Pearson's correlation coefficient was calculated between the tension and misfit variables for all the groups evaluated in the study. Table 3 and figure 23 show that there was a positive correlation (p<0.0074) between tension values and marginal misfit. This positive correlation was considered strong (r=0.4169).

Table 3. Correlation of the marginal misfit values with the stress values induced in the superstructure.

	Pearson's coefficient	(P)
Values of Mismatches/Values of Tensions	de 0,4169	< 0,0074

Pearson's coefficient (-1 to 1)

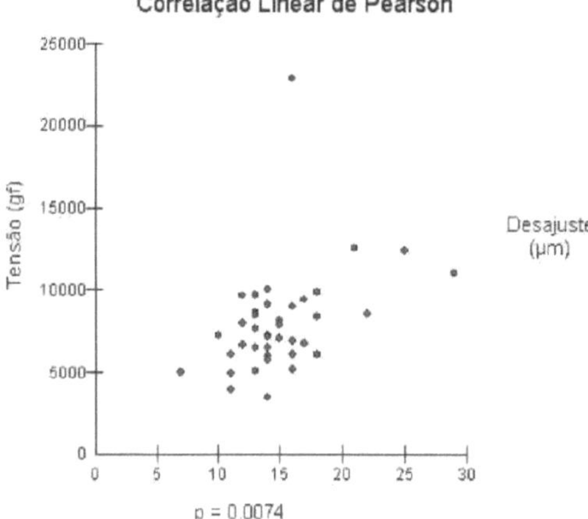

Figura 23   Correlation of all misalignments/all marginal misalignment voltages with the induced voltage values.

It can be said that when there is an increase in marginal misalignment values, there is also an increase in tension values.

6. Discussion

The first hypothesis proposed by this study, that a transfer molding technique using a new material would be better than existing ones, was rejected. The technique that had the best results of the four studied was the one that used prefabricated sticks of chemically activated acrylic resin for splinting. The results show that the group that used the new material to splint the transfers did not lead to a significant reduction in the stress values induced in the superstructure.

According to Sahin & Çehreli, 2001 one of the main challenges for a prosthodontist is to deliver an acceptable prosthesis that does not compromise the longevity of the treatment. Passive fit (synonymous with "ideal fit") is assumed to be one of the most significant prerequisites for maintaining the bone-implant interface. To provide passive fit or a stress-free suprastructure, the structure should theoretically induce zero stress on the implant components and the surrounding bone. This requirement can be met by complete and simultaneous contact of the inner surfaces of all the retainers by all the abutments. Undoubtedly, the precise reproduction of the position of the implants for working models plays a significant role. In addition, according to Phillips, *et al.,* 1994, an impression technique should ideally take the shortest time, be easy to perform, inexpensive, comfortable for the patient and provide the best results.

In this context, although the techniques did not differ statistically in terms of marginal misalignments (the lowest average was obtained in Group C, 14μm - squares splinted with resin rods), averages lower than the average of other studies, these misalignments induced tension in the superstructure.

The technique that had the best results of the four studied, however, took the longest to perform, requiring several procedural steps, operative difficulty and discomfort for the patient. The technique that used a new material did not differ from the others in terms of marginal mismatches. With regard to tensions, except for   except for the square transfer technique with resin rods, there was no statistically significant difference either. The advantages of this technique over the others are: shorter execution time (executed in a single step), ease of operation, low cost and patient comfort.

The techniques tested in this study have been commonly used in clinical practice and have also been the subject of many studies to assess their accuracy. However, most of these experiments used microscopy as the measurement method, while others used extensometry, finite element and photoelasticity. No study has used two measurement methods simultaneously, as reported in the literature: Using resin rods to join the transfers (Humphries *et al.,* 1990; Carr and Sokol, 19991; Fenton *et al.,* 1991; Rodney et al., 1991; Assif *et al.,*1992; Carr, 1992; Phillips et *al.,* 1994; Pinto et *al.,* 2001; Goiato *et al.,* 2002; Assunçao, et *al.,* 2004;Rodrigues, 2006; Del'Acqua, *et al.,* 2008; Gennari Filho *et al.* 2009); using acrylic resin over dental floss to bond the transfers (Spector *et al.,* 1990; Hsu et *al.,* 1993; Inturregui et *al.,* 1993; Assif *et al.,* 1996; Burawi et al., 1997; Conrad *et al.,* 2009); using acrylic resin and self-curing composite resin (Augustin *et al.,* 2009); using light-curing composite resin (Ivanhoe, *et al.,* 2006); using plaster for molding (Inturregui et al., 1993; Assif, *et al.,* 1999; Wise, 1991); conical and square isolated (Carr and Sokol, 1991; Carr, 1991; Carr, 1992; Rodney et *al.,* 1991).

When the positioning of the analogues in the specimens is evaluated microscopically only in the horizontal plane (Rodney, Johansen, Harris, 1991; Liou *et al.,* 1993; Pinto, 1995; Goiato, 1997; Burawi, *et al.,* 1997; Del'Acqua *et al.,* 2008), the results are less accurate, since the precision and inaccuracy of the transfer techniques are three-dimensional.

Few studies incorporate electrical resistance extensometers as a measurement method to determine which technique introduces the least distortion (Inturregui *et al.,* 1993; Assif, Marshak, Schimidt, 1996; Assif *et al.,* 1999; Nissan et al., 2001; Naconecy *et al.,* 2004). Extensometry enables exercises such as the comparison of stresses resulting from the tightening of one (according to the protocol for the laboratory evaluation of passivity using the single screw test) or two prosthetic screws (reproducing the clinical situation when prostheses are installed).

Other methods for analyzing stresses, such as photoelasticity and the finite element, are limited to the analysis of a single prosthetic structure (Koke *et al.,* 2004), and do not allow for quantitative evaluation of the data.

Extensometry was the method of choice in this study for evaluating induced tensions, as its reliability is respected in the literature. It also enabled quantitative evaluation of the data.

Several studies have demonstrated the use of the method in quantitative tests (Glantz *et al,* 1993*;* Watanabe *et al,* 2000*;* Naconecy *et al,* 2004; Tramontino *et al,* 2008; Daroz 2009).

The amount of deformation suffered by a specimen measured by a strain gauge model depends on a number of variables such as: the magnitude and direction of the imposed load, the design of the specimen, the material of the specimen and its modulus of elasticity, the position of the strain gauges on the surface of the specimen (Daroz, 2009), the perfect bonding of the strain gauges, the correct calibration of the measuring device, the torquing performed for the model readings (even with a calibrated torque wrench), the loss of preload due to plastic deformation of the fixing prosthetic screws caused by repeated torquing, among others.

The second hypothesis of this study, that there would be a direct correlation between marginal misfit and the tensions generated, was confirmed. Pearson's coefficient between the variables **tension** and **misfit** for all the groups evaluated was r=0.4169 with p<0.0074, indicating that there was a positive correlation, i.e. when there is an increase in marginal misfit values, there is also an increase in tension values. This correlation was considered to be strong, given that perfect correlation occurs when the coefficient is equal to 1. The proportionality between the variables was also confirmed. This observation is in line with the results of Daroz, 2009, who, when evaluating axial and lateral tensions generated by different patterns of marginal misfit in implant-retained multiple structures, found that higher levels of misfit produced greater amounts of tension.

Other studies that found a direct relationship between marginal misfit and induced stress (Clelland, 1995; Millington & Leung, 1995) concluded that there was no proportionality between the variables. However, the results presented by Torres, (2005), and Tramontino (2008), showed that there was no correlation between the values of marginal adaptation and the stresses generated by the implants.

The methodology employed in the experiment, using two measurement methods, allowed a more complete view of the various techniques studied, thus enabling a better assessment of what can occur in a clinical situation. The results also showed that although the misalignment values were small, lower than the average of other studies, these misalignments still induced tension in the suprastructure. The search for new impression techniques and new materials could be the subject of further research.

7. Conclusion

Within the limitations of this study, it was possible to conclude that:

1-   Of the four techniques studied, the most accurate was the one that used square transfers splinted with prefabricated resin rods, for both misfit and induced tension;

2-   Há direct correlation between marginal misfit and stress generated in the superstructure.

8. References *

1.	Abdullah MA, Talic YF. The effect of custom tray material type and fabrication technique on tensile bond strength of impression material adhesive systems. J. Oral Rehabil. 2003; 30(3): 312-317.

2.	Aparicio CA New method to routinely achieve passive fit of ceramometal prostheses over Branemark Osseointegrated implants: A two-year report. Int. J. Periodontics Restorative Dent. 1994; 14(5): 405-419.

3.	Assif D, Fenton A, Zarb G, Schimitt A. Comparative accuracy of implant impression procedures. Int. J. Periodontics Restorative Dent. 1992; 12(2): 11221.

4.	Assif D, Marshak B, Nissan JA. modified impression technique for implant- supported restoration. J. Prosthet. Dent. 1994; 71(6): 589-591.

5.	Assif D, Marshak B, Schmidt. A. Accuracy of implant impression techniques. Int. J. Oral Maxillofac. Implants.1996; 11(2):216-222.

6.	Assif D, Nissan J, Varsano I, Singer A. Accuracy of implant impression splinted techniques: Effect of splinting material. Int. J. Oral Maxillofac. Implants. 1999; 14(6): 885-888.

7.	Assunçâo WG, Gennari Filho H, Zaniquelli O. Evaluation of transfer impressions for osseointegrated implants at various angulations. Implant Dent. 2004; 13(4): 358-366.

8.	Alves Junior RT, Gouveia CVD, Carvalho WR, Ferreira VF, Mussallen FO, Barbosa ESP. New impression technique with acrylic resin coping bonding compared to transfer with silicone adhesive. Braz Oral Res 2009;23(Suppl. 1):92-110 (Proceedings of the 26th SBPqO Annual Meeting); Aguas de Lindoia - Sao Paulo - Brazil.

9.	Augustin A, Flamia KS, Manfro R, Bortoluzzi MC. Evaluation of polymerization contraction of Sterngold resin. Braz Oral Res 2009;23(Suppl. 1):92-110 (Proceedings of the 26th SBPqO Annual Meeting); Aguas de Lindoia - Sao Paulo - Brazil

10.	Adell R, Lekholm U, Rockler B, Branemark PI. A 15-year study of osseointegrated implants in the treatment of the edentulous jaw. Int J Oral Surg. 1981; 10(6):387- 416.

11.	Bauman GR, Mills M, Rapley JW, Hallmon WW. Plaque-induced inflammation around implants. Int J Oral Maxillofac Implants. 1992; 7(3):330-7.

---

*According to the UNICAMP/FOP standard, based on the International Committee of Medical Journal Editors - Vancouver Group standard. Journal abbreviations in accordance with Medline.

12.   Bindra B, Heath JR. Adhesion of elastomeric impression materials to trays. J. Oral Rehabil. 1997; 24(1): 63-69.

13.   Burawi, G, Houston F, Byrne D, Claffey N. A comparison of the dimensional accuracy of the splinted and unsplinted impression techniques for the BoneLock implant system. J. Prosthet. Dent. 1997; 77(1): 68-75.

14.   Bressani JA. Comparative analysis of single implant transfer molding accuracy between irreversible hydrocolloid and silicone adhesive [dissertation] Campinas: Sao Leopoldo Mandic; 2006

15.   Carr AB. A comparison of impression techniques for a five-implant mandibular model. Int. J. Oral Maxillofac. Implants.1991; 6(4): 448-455.

16.   Carr AB. Comparison of impression techniques for a two-implant 15-degree divergent model. Int. J. Oral Maxillofac. Implants. 1992; 7(4): 468-475.

17.   Carr AB, Sokol J. Accuracy of casts produced by the Nobelpharma impression techniques.[Abstract 198] J Dent Res 1991; 290.

18.   Cheshire PD, Hobkirk JA. An in vivo quantitative analysis of the fit of Nobel Biocare implant superstructures. J. Oral Rehabil. 1996; 23(11): 782-789.

19.   Coelho AB. Evaluation of the morphodimensional behavior of impression materials used in dental implants. [dissertation]: Bauru: USP/FOB; 1997.

20.   Cabral LM. Comparative analysis of four implant molding techniques. [dissertation] Brasilia: UNB/ FCS; 2005.

21.   Chavez AM. Evaluation of the accuracy of molding techniques for implant-supported prostheses on aligned implants and non-aligned implants. [dissertation]: Araraquara: UNESP/FOAR; 2007.

22.   Conrad HJ, Pesun IJ, DeLong R, Hodges JS. Accuracy of two impression techniques with angulated implants. J. Prosthet. Dent. 2007; 97(6): 349-356.

23.   Daoudi MF, Setchell DJ, Searson LJ. A laboratory investigation of the accuracy of two impression techniques for single-tooth implants. Int. J. Prosthodont. 2001; 14(2): 152-158.

24.   Daroz LGD. Mechanical behavior of multiple implant-retained restorations in the presence of marginal misalignments. [thesis] Piracicaba: UNICAMP/FOP; 2009.

25.   De La Cruz JE, Frankenbusch PD, Ercoli C, Moss ME, Craser GN, Tallents RH.

Verification jig for implant-supported prostheses: A comparison of standard impressions with verification jigs made of different materials. J. Prosthet. Dent. 2002; 88(3):329-336.

26. Del'Acqua MA, Arioli-Filho JN, Campagnoni MA, De Assis Mollo JRF. Accuracy of impression and pouring techniques for an implant-supported prosthesis. International Journal of Oral Maxillofacial Implants. 2008; 23(2): 226-236.

27. Dumbrigue HB, Gurun DC, Javid NS. Prefabricated acrylic resin bars for splinting implant transfer copings. J. Prosthet. Dent. 2000; 84(1): 108-110.

28. Fenton AH. The accuracy of implant impression procedures. J Dent Res. 1991; 70:399.

29. Goiato MC, Domitti SS, Consani S. Influence of impression materials and implant transfer techniques on the dimensional accuracy of plaster models. Jbc: J. Bras. Odontol. Clin. 1998; 2(8): 45-50.

30. Goiato MC, Gennari Filho H, Fajardo RS, Assunçâo WG, Dekon SFC... Comparison of three impression materials and three transfer molding techniques for implants. Bci: Rev. Bras. Cir. Implantodont. 2002; 9(34): 164-168.

31. Gregory-Head B, Labarre E. Two-step pick-up impression procedure for implant-retained overdentures. J Prosthet Dent. 1999; 82(5): 615-616.

32. Gennari Filho H, Mazaro VQ, Vedovato E, Assunçâo WG, Dos Santos PH. Accuracy of impression techniques for implants. Prt 2 - Comparison of Splintig. J.of Prosthodont. 2009; 18 172-176.

33. Herbst D, Nel Jc, Driessen CH, Becker PJ. Evaluation of impression accuracy for osseointegrated implant supported superstructures. J. Prosthet. Dent. 2000; 83(5): 555-561.

34. Hsu CC, Millstein PL, Stein RS. A comparative analysis of the accuracy of implant transfer techniques. J. Prosthet. Dent. 1993; 69(6): 588-593.

35. Humphries, R. M.; Yaman, P.; Bloem, T. J. The accuracy of implant master casts constructed from transfer impressions. Int. J. Oral Maxillofac. Implants. 1990; 5(4): 331-336.

36. Hussaini S, Wong T. One clinical visit for a multiple implant restoration master cast fabrication. J. Prosthet. Dent. 1997; 78(6): 550-553.

37. Inturregui JA, Aquilino AS, Ryther JS, Lund PS. Evaluation of three impression techniques for osseointegrated oral implants. J. Prosthet. Dent. 1993; 69(5): 503-509.

38. Ivanhoe JR, Adrian ED, Krantz WA, Edge MJ. An impression technique for osseointegrated implants. J. Prosthet. Dent. 1991; 66(3): 410-411.

39. Jemt T. Failures and complications in 391 consecutively inserted fixed prostheses supported by Branemark implants in edentulous jaws: A study of treatment from the time of prosthesis placement to the first annual checkup. Int. J. Oral Maxillofac. Implants. 1991; 6(3): 270-276.

40. Kallus T, Bessing C. Loose gold screws frequently occur in full-arch fixed prostheses supported by osseointegrated implants after 5 years. Int. J. Oral Maxillofac. Implants. 1994; 9(2): 169-178.

41. Kim S, Nicholls JI, Han CH, Lee KW. Displacement of implant components from impressions to definitive casts. Int J Oral Maxillofac Implants. 2006; 21:747-55.

42. Lee HS, Hochsteller JL, Ercoli C. The accuracy of implants impressions: A systematic review. J. Prosthet. Dent. 2008; 100(4): 285-291.

43. Lorenzoni M, Pertl C, Penkner K, Polansky R, Sedaj B, WegscheiderWA. Comparison of the transfer precision of three different impression materials in combination with transfer caps for the Frialit® -2 system. J. Oral Rehabil. 2000; 27(7): 629-638.

44. Lopes Junior T. Determination of the forces generated by chemically activated acrylic resins during the implant position transfer process - Photoelastic analysis [dissertation] Uberlandia: UFU/Odontologia; 2008.

45. Luebke RJ, Scandrett FR, Kerber PE. The effect of delayed and second pours on elastomeric impression material accuracy. J. Prosthet. Dent. 1979; 41(5): 517-521.

46. Millington ND, Leung T. Inaccurate fit of implant superstructures. Part I: stresses generated on the superstructure relative to size of fit discrepancy. Int J Prosthodont. 1995;8(6):511-516

47. McCartney JW, Pearson R. Segmental framework matrix: Master cast verification, corrected cast guide, and analog transfer template for implant- supported prostheses. J. Prosthet. Dent. 1994; 71(2): 197-200.

48. Mojon P, Oberholzer JP, Meyer JM, Belser UC. Polymerization shrinkage of index and pattern acrylic resins. J. Prosthet. Dent. 1990; 64(6): 684-688.

49. Moon PC, Eshleman JR, Douglas HB, Garrett SG. Comparison of accuracy of soldering indices for fixed prostheses. J. Prosthet. Dent. 1978; 40(1): 35-38.

50. Modesto LCP. *In vitro* comparison of the accuracy of models obtained from the

transfer molding of implant-supported prostheses, using a silicone and a polyether.[dissertation] Campinas: Sâo Leopoldo Mandic; 2006.

51. Naconecy MM, Teixeira ER, Shinkai RS, Frasca LC, Carvieri A. Evaluation of the accuracy of 3 transfer techniques for implant-supported prostheses with multiple abutments. Int. J. Oral Maxillofac. Implants. 2004; 19(2): 192-198.

52. Ness EM, Nicholls JI, Rubenstein JE, Smith DE. Accuracy of the acrylic resin pattern for the implant-retained prosthesis. Int. J. Prosthodont.1992; 5(6): 542-549.

53. Naert I, Quirynen M, van Steenberghe D, Darius P. A study of 589 consecutive implants supporting complete fixed prostheses . Part II: Prosthetic aspects . J Prosthet Dent. 1992; 68(6):949-56.

54. Nissan J, Laufer BZ, Brosh T, Assif D. Accuracy of three polyvinyl siloxane putty-wash impression techniques. J. Prosthet. Dent.2000; 83(2): 161-165.

55. Nissan J, Gross M, Shifman A, Assif D. Effect of wash bulk on the accuracy of polyvinyl siloxane putty-wash impressions. J. Oral Rehabil. 2002; 29(4): 357361.

56. Nissan J, Barnea E, Krauze E, Assif D. Impression technique for partially edentulous patients. J. Prosthet. Dent. 2002; 88(1): 103-104.

57. Phillips K M. The accuracy of three implant impression techniques: A three-dimensional analysis. Int. J. Oral Maxillofac. Implants. 1994; 9(5): 533-540.

58. Pinto JHN. Comparative study between molding techniques for dental implants. Rev. Fac. Odontol. Bauru, Bauru. 2001; 93/4): 167-172.

59. Ribas FL. Comparative analysis of five different implant prosthesis molding techniques. [dissertation] Belo Horizonte: PUC/Odontologia; 2008.

60. Rodney J, Johansen R, Harris W. Dimensional accuracy of two implant impression copings. [Abstract 953]. J Dent Res 1991;70:385.

61. Romero GG Engelmeier R, Powers JM, Canterbury AA. Accuracy of three corrective techniques for implant bar fabrication. J. Prosthet. Dent. 2000; 84(6): 602-607.

62. Rodrigues RA. *In vitro* evaluation of different techniques and methods for joining impression transfers used in implant dentistry [dissertation] Natal: Univ.Potiguar/Odontologia; 2006.

63. Sahin S, Çehreli MC. The significance of passive framework fit in implant prosthodontics: Current status. Implant. Dent. 2001; 10(2): 85-92.

64. Shiau JC, Chen LL, Wu CT. An accurate impression method for implant prosthesis fabrication. J. Prosthet. Dent. 1994; 72(1): 23-25.

65. Skalak R. Biomechanical considerations in osseointegrated prostheses. J. Prosthet. Dent. 1993; 49(6): 843-848.

66. Sakuno A. Analysis of the accuracy of two molding techniques for prostheses on implants[dissertation] Campinas: Sao Leopoldo mandic; 2004.

67. Spector MR, Donovan TE, Nicholls JI. An evaluation of impression techniques for osseointegrated implants. J. Prosthet. Dent. 1990; 63(4): 444447.

68. Tramontino VS. Implant-retained fixed prostheses: influence of the intermediate abutment and ceramic cooking cycles on the misalignments and stresses induced in the fixtures. [Piracicaba: UNICAMP/FOP; 2008.

69. Vigolo P, Majzoub Z, Cordioli G. In vitro comparison of master cast accuracy for single-tooth implant replacement. J. Prosthet. Dent. 2000; 83(5): 562-566.

70. Vigolo P, Majzoub Z, Cordioli G. Evaluation of the accuracy of three techniques used for multiple implant abutment impressions. J. Prosthet. Dent. 2003; 89(2): 186-192.

71. Zarb GA, Schmitt A. Osseointegration and the endentulous predicament. The 10-year-old Toronto study. Br Dent J. 1991;170(12):439-44.

72. Waskewicz GA. Ostrowski JS, Parks VJ. Photoelastic analysis of stress distribution transmitted from a fixed prosthesis attached to osseointegrated implants. Int. J. Oral Maxillofac. Implants. 1994; 9(4): 405-411.

73. Wee AG. Comparison of impression materials for direct multi-implant impressions. J. Prosthet. Dent. 2000; 83(3): 323-331.

74. Wise M. Fit of implant-supported fixed prostheses fabricated on master casts made from a dental stone and a dental plaster. J. Prosthet. Dent. 2001; 86(5): 532-538.

9. Appendix

Original data - Voltage Models

Group	Model	Handle	Reading	Repeat 1	Repeat 2	Repeat 3	Average piece
Group A	1	A	AB	5172,12	5265,72	5379,84	8532,96
			BA	5388,05	4855,70	5479,97	
		B	AB	11931,40	12187,90	12129,20	
			BA	11751,00	11087,20	11767,40	
	2	A	AB	9251,40	7212,29	8116,92	7255,13
			BA	7387,17	7190,97	7293,75	
		B	AB	6820,20	6663,09	6640,56	
			BA	6936,35	6609,41	6939,44	
	3	A	AB	2158,46	2084,26	2190,07	7256,15
			BA	1881,38	1953,28	2069,67	
		B	AB	12576,90	12413,90	12458,90	
			BA	12587,20	12307,30	12392,50	
	4	A	AB	12995,90	12904,70	12859,30	7675,09
			BA	13319,50	13365,20	13496,40	
		B	AB	1721,05	1835,13	1748,13	
			BA	2672,79	2550,28	2632,68	
	5	A	AB	11553,80	11710,50	11720,30	12456,28
			BA	12264,90	12476,80	12486,60	
		B	AB	13094,40	13373,60	13396,80	
			BA	12385,90	12398,20	12613,50	
	6	A	AB	7804,74	7359,00	8255,54	8623,12
			BA	8734,19	8907,67	8850,72	
		B	AB	9741,80	9559,57	10388,80	
			BA	1088,90	11275,80	11510,70	
	7	A	AB	14093,80	14488,00	14312,50	9732,96
			BA	15339,10	15156,60	15349,60	
		B	AB	4595,34	4163,08	4185,10	
			BA	5249,57	4827,80	5035,08	
	8	A	AB	15487,50	15064,10	14967,30	9421,77
			BA	15925,40	16627,10	15926,40	
		B	AB	3776,73	4385,04	4006,44	
			BA	2778,60	1985,32	2131,31	
	9	A	AB	6337,55	6353,22	6404,06	9145,37
			BA	5907,92	5966,07	5789,91	
		B	AB	11989,10	11948,50	12037,50	
			BA	12566,00	12223,40	12221,20	
	10	A	AB	2764,84	2991,27	2808,25	3492,64
			BA	3160,68	3297,09	3145,81	
		B	AB	3806,02	3828,97	3847,93	
			BA	4161,28	4072,69	4026,89	
	Average gf (Group A)				8359,15		8359,15
	DP				4462,26		2287,82

Group	Model	Handle	Reading	Repeat 1	Repeat 2	Repeat 3	Average piece
Group B	1	A	AB	1970,96	2193,47	1958,67	8156,07
			BA	1263,66	1327,90	1450,72	
		B	AB	14261,00	13856,40	14283,30	
			BA	15263,30	15115,00	14928,40	
	2	A	AB	7432,15	7403,87	7944,66	8418,71
			BA	7085,75	6740,54	7255,99	
		B	AB	8566,41	9056,32	9234,80	
			BA	10533,30	8876,67	10894,10	
	3	A	AB	2161,12	1767,02	2172,54	6036,70
			BA	2021,82	2171,99	2235,12	
		B	AB	9840,64	10088,00	9838,92	
			BA	9965,10	9985,50	10192,60	
	4	A	AB	1387,81	1597,90	1593,30	6897,75
			BA	2036,94	2056,14	2139,53	
		B	AB	11774,30	11821,70	11982,00	
			BA	12184,20	12019,50	12179,70	
	5	A	AB	6589,48	6864,60	7264,05	12586,43
			BA	7009,01	6763,98	7176,69	
		B	AB	18165,90	18307,60	18148,90	
			BA	18202,00	18099,30	18445,60	
	6	A	AB	3550,07	3767,90	3797,50	6678,48
			BA	3374,41	3164,96	3271,40	
		B	AB	9894,64	9671,96	9773,98	
			BA	9845,08	10048,50	9981,36	
	7	A	AB	3170,62	2886,19	3373,50	7968,75
			BA	3047,51	3125,53	2988,11	
		B	AB	13022,60	12729,00	12684,20	
			BA	12655,50	12973,80	12968,40	

Group	Model	Handle	Reading	Repeat 1	Repeat 2	Repeat 3	Average piece
	8	A	AB	10231,00	10232,20	10128,70	9661,99
			BA	9797,06	9749,94	9708,96	
		B	AB	9328,71	9091,70	9214,81	
			BA	9558,90	9353,57	9548,35	
	9	A	AB	31581,30	30926,20	37839,60	22904,05
			BA	31723,30	13080,60	41198,00	
		B	AB	11015,20	13617,30	16059,30	
			BA	16924,40	14448,80	16434,60	
	10	A	AB	11951,00	12201,60	11875,80	11067,37
			BA	9826,55	9066,22	8874,34	
		B	AB	11211,20	11202,10	11026,10	
			BA	12493,50	11397,80	11682,25	
Average gf(Group B)				10037,63			10037,63
DP				6966,58			4953,50

Group	Model	Handle	Reading	Repeat 1	Repeat 2	Repeat 3	Average piece
	1	A	AB	313,97	94,36	25,35	4919,85
			BA	384,96	478,38	438,33	
		B	AB	9494,66	9470,34	9381,79	
			BA	9754,69	9670,40	9530,91	
	2	A	AB	557,56	771,50	628,62	5078,25
			BA	1330,97	1085,23	1368,68	
		B	AB	9014,99	9198,09	9165,69	
			BA	9343,75	9097,94	9375,93	
	3	A	AB	1003,65	1228,69	1155,90	5776,28
			BA	947,68	1046,16	904,28	
		B	AB	10682,20	10591,30	10486,80	
			BA	10256,80	10610,20	10401,70	
	4	A	AB	1638,78	1483,03	1429,25	6482,13
			BA	2333,99	2224,08	2278,82	
		B	AB	11134,60	11060,50	10950,50	
			BA	11143,80	10946,80	11161,40	
	5	A	AB	5354,49	5641,54	5322,85	7029,96
			BA	7011,89	6861,18	7377,71	
		B	AB	6959,62	7231,26	7233,31	
			BA	8489,09	8142,49	8734,08	
	6	A	AB	2290,82	2304,34	2282,54	7071,38
			BA	2758,68	2673,26	2919,06	
		B	AB	11405,40	11353,50	11579,80	
			BA	11865,60	11454,00	11969,60	
	7	A	AB	781,00	833,34	623,40	6093,45
			BA	199,05	400,41	117,56	
		B	AB	11614,00	11314,20	11613,10	
			BA	11840,70	11768,00	12016,60	
	8	A	AB	1031,62	1113,19	1190,76	6058,21
			BA	719,56	662,52	567,03	
		B	AB	11368,10	11157,00	11237,10	
			BA	11099,90	11204,40	11347,30	
	9	A	AB	3611,09	3484,14	3246,15	6064,66
			BA	3007,52	2927,33	2993,80	
		B	AB	8772,28	8728,64	8776,16	
			BA	9080,81	9028,18	9119,79	
	10	A	AB	3644,09	3534,87	3099,10	3932,43
			BA	3655,23	3826,94	3929,41	
		B	AB	4076,79	4166,60	3894,87	
			BA	4215,73	4708,23	4437,32	
Mean (Group C) SD				5850,66			5850,66
				4248,25			976,14

Group	Model	Handle	Reading	Repeat 1	Repeat 2	Repeat 3	Average piece
Group D	1	A	AB	454,58	635,78	226,11	5013,82
			BA	877,05	1319,06	1112,22	
		B	AB	9081,82	9470,33	8739,80	
			BA	9441,28	9554,77	9253,04	
	2	A	AB	2014,49	2055,52	1798,49	6762,81
			BA	2308,82	2445,42	2304,27	
		B	AB	11270,20	11249,30	11097,20	
			BA	11833,60	11241,10	11535,30	
	3	A	AB	2508,55	2494,85	2774,08	7154,81
			BA	2901,11	2383,95	2256,37	
		B	AB	11709,10	11709,60	11740,10	
			BA	11707,00	11710,90	11962,10	
	4	A	AB	1637,67	1482,76	1428,86	6481,97
			BA	2333,79	2224,22	2278,84	
		B	AB	11134,50	11061,40	10950,50	

			Face				average
			BA	11143,70	10946,60	11160,80	
	5	A	AB	302,10	483,63	355,76	5195,74
			BA	1716,40	2011,73	2218,16	
		B	AB	9303,71	9204,57	8998,42	
			BA	8858,39	9595,69	9300,30	
	6	A	AB	2568,56	2470,29	2426,62	8470,44
			BA	3689,78	3361,30	3476,24	
		B	AB	13439,70	13444,70	13533,80	
			BA	14752,00	13996,90	14485,40	
	7	A	AB	4121,73	3615,57	3831,92	10017,93
			BA	3461,42	3936,07	3652,71	
		B	AB	16436,40	16138,40	16365,90	
			BA	15859,80	16680,40	16114,80	
	8	A	AB	4921,16	3825,77	4021,87	9900,22
			BA	3925,57	4043,47	3970,68	
		B	AB	16560,70	14408,60	15997,30	
			BA	15210,70	16268,20	15648,60	
	9	A	AB	4224,37	4084,03	3946,91	7897,71
			BA	4457,80	4425,37	4405,86	
		B	AB	11595,30	11386,50	11443,00	
			BA	11542,50	11584,30	11676,60	
	10	A	AB	4637,93	4792,76	4709,69	9012,92
			BA	5132,15	4958,45	4932,40	
		B	AB	13065,30	13190,10	13014,30	
			BA	13489,10	13310,80	12922,00	
Average gf(Group D)					7590,84		7590,84
DP					5124,18		1782,54

1.2 Mismatch - Models

Group	Model	Face	Pillar A (mm)			Pillar B (mm)			C-pillar (mm)			average
MATRIX SCT	1	V	0,018	0,015	0,019	0,008	0,010	0,011	0,010	0,014	0,009	0,012
		L	0,017	0,020	0,016	0,011	0,009	0,009	0,010	0,007	0,011	
MATRIX T	1	V	0,046	0,040	0,046	0,010	0,012	0,013	0,017	0,012	0,014	0,022
		L	0,020	0,022	0,018	0,031	0,030	0,027	0,012	0,012	0,013	

Group	Model	Face	Pillar A (mm)			Pillar B (mm)			C-pillar (mm)			average	GA AVERAGE
Group A	1	V	0,019	0,020	0,018	0,017	0,019	0,015	0,014	0,013	0,015	0,022	0,016
		L	0,015	0,018	0,015	0,060	0,050	0,051	0,012	0,018	0,013		median
	2	V	0,016	0,018	0,017	0,006	0,008	0,008	0,009	0,011	0,009	0,010	0,014
		L	0,004	0,002	0,004	0,014	0,013	0,016	0,009	0,009	0,011		
	3	V	0,018	0,015	0,020	0,014	0,011	0,013	0,014	0,012	0,012	0,014	
		L	0,010	0,012	0,011	0,011	0,010	0,013	0,020	0,015	0,015		
	4	V	0,011	0,013	0,014	0,016	0,014	0,014	0,017	0,015	0,014	0,013	
		L	0,015	0,014	0,013	0,015	0,016	0,013	0,008	0,009	0,007		
	5	V	0,082	0,.081	0,084	0,014	0,017	0,016	0,020	0,015	0,021	0,025	
		L	0,019	0,020	0,018	0,019	0,016	0,018	0,020	0,017	0,016		
	6	V	0,014	0,016	0,015	0,011	0,009	0,011	0,014	0,011	0,013	0,013	
		L	0,015	0,015	0,012	0,015	0,016	0,014	0,009	0,010	0,012		
	7	V	0,013	0,016	0,014	0,009	0,011	0,012	0,026	0,019	0,023	0,013	
		L	0,010	0,009	0,011	0,011	0,013	0,012	0,009	0,009	0,011		
	8	V	0,032	0,033	0,031	0,012	0,011	0,011	0,031	0,025	0,023	0,017	
		L	0,012	0,008	0,012	0,011	0,009	0,008	0,016	0,015	0,014		
	9	V	0,017	0,015	0,020	0,018	0,018	0,020	0,016	0,018	0,017	0,014	
		L	0,010	0,015	0,010	0,010	0,011	0,013	0,013	0,010	0,009		
	10	V	0,015	0,016	0,014	0,011	0,012	0,010	0,014	0,013	0,015	0,014	
		L	0,009	0,010	0,012	0,018	0,020	0,021	0,011	0,011	0,012		

Group	Model	Face	Pillar A (mm)			Pillar B (mm)			C-pillar (mm)			average	GB AVERAGE
Group B	1	V	0,016	0,016	0,018	0,019	0,022	0,017	0,020	0,021	0,021	0,015	0,026
		L	0,009	0,008	0,010	0,013	0,011	0,013	0,010	0,013	0,011		mrdiana
	2	V	0,014	0,016	0,015	0,015	0,017	0,013	0,014	0,016	0,015	0,018	0,015
		L	0,018	0,016	0,015	0,032	0,033	0,031	0,013	0,014	0,013		
	3	V	0,016	0,014	0,015	0,013	0,015	0,013	0,017	0,014	0,016	0,014	
		L	0,012	0,011	0,015	0,011	0,015	0,013	0,012	0,011	0,014		
	4	V	0,018	0,016	0,017	0,019	0,014	0,013	0,017	0,020	0,018	0,016	
		L	0,009	0,009	0,011	0,021	0,020	0,021	0,016	0,014	0,014		
	5	V	0,018	0,015	0,016	0,013	0,013	0,016	0,017	0,011	0,015	0,021	
		L	0,017	0,016	0,016	0,049	0,048	0,052	0,017	0,016	0,018		
	6	V	0,012	0,011	0,010	0,016	0,011	0,012	0,017	0,016	0,017	0,012	
		L	0,012	0,010	0,012	0,013	0,011	0,012	0,008	0,009	0,010		
	7	V	0,017	0,015	0,016	0,010	0,012	0,011	0,011	0,010	0,014	0,012	
		L	0,013	0,014	0,014	0,013	0,013	0,014	0,007	0,009	0,008		
	8	V	0,017	0,014	0,015	0,014	0,013	0,011	0,018	0,011	0,012	0,012	
		L	0,009	0,011	0,012	0,013	0,014	0,010	0,011	0,008	0,011		
	9	V	0,016	0,014	0,014	0,088	0,091	0,090	0,014	0,016	0,018	0,115	
		L	0,058	0,052	0,051	0,381	0,386	0,383	0,132	0,131	0,128		
	10	V	0,015	0,016	0,014	0,015	0,012	0,014	0,011	0,010	0,008	0,029	
		L	0,008	0,007	0,011	0,112	0,109	0,106	0,017	0,016	0,018		

Group	Model	Face	Pillar A (mm)			Pillar B (mm)			C-pillar (mm)			average	AVERAGE CG
Group C	1	V	0,015	0,010	0,014	0,009	0,006	0,008	0,006	0,010	0,008	0,011	0,014
		L	0,011	0,010	0,008	0,017	0,016	0,018	0,008	0,011	0,009		median
	2	V	0,016	0,014	0,018	0,010	0,011	0,010	0,018	0,017	0,019	0,013	0,014
		L	0,013	0,012	0,014	0,009	0,010	0,011	0,011	0,010	0,013		
	3	V	0,017	0,016	0,016	0,010	0,008	0,011	0,020	0,018	0,016	0,014	
		L	0,013	0,015	0,015	0,018	0,014	0,016	0,011	0,011	0,012		
	4	V	0,009	0,008	0,008	0,015	0,012	0,015	0,020	0,014	0,018	0,014	
		L	0,016	0,014	0,013	0,013	0,012	0,014	0,020	0,015	0,015		
	5	V	0,024	0,023	0,022	0,011	0,011	0,012	0,018	0,016	0,019	0,015	
		L	0,015	0,014	0,012	0,010	0,012	0,015	0,013	0,010	0,011		
	6	V	0,020	0,019	0,018	0,013	0,013	0,015	0,016	0,011	0,014	0,015	
		L	0,013	0,016	0,016	0,015	0,014	0,016	0,015	0,013	0,012		
	7	V	0,018	0,019	0,020	0,009	0,009	0,010	0,020	0,018	0,017	0,016	
		L	0,017	0,014	0,017	0,020	0,017	0,020	0,018	0,017	0,016		
	8	V	0,014	0,013	0,016	0,011	0,011	0,010	0,013	0,008	0,012	0,011	
		L	0,014	0,012	0,010	0,011	0,009	0,012	0,007	0,008	0,010		
	9	V	0,019	0,020	0,019	0,014	0,017	0,016	0,030	0,028	0,024	0,018	

Group	Model	Face	Pillar A (mm)			Pillar B (mm)			C-pillar (mm)			average	GD AVERAGE
		L	0,018	0,016	0,019	0,017	0,018	0,019	0,011	0,012	0,010		
	10	V	0,008	0,007	0,009	0,008	0,009	0,008	0,012	0,010	0,014	0,011	
		L	0,014	0,012	0,012	0,023	0,020	0,018	0,005	0,005	0,004		
Group D	1	V	0,006	0,005	0,006	0,013	0,009	0,011	0,007	0,008	0,009	0,007	0,014
		L	0,006	0,008	0,006	0,006	0,008	0,006	0,007	0,006	0,004		median
	2	V	0,018	0,019	0,017	0,018	0,017	0,016	0,020	0,017	0,018	0,017	0,015
		L	0,018	0,016	0,017	0,021	0,018	0,017	0,010	0,011	0,009		
	3	V	0,020	0,021	0,019	0,014	0,012	0,013	0,017	0,015	0,018	0,014	
		L	0,011	0,009	0,010	0,011	0,013	0,016	0,010	0,013	0,011		
	4	V	0,011	0,012	0,014	0,020	0,017	0,017	0,015	0,012	0,013	0,013	
		L	0,012	0,010	0,011	0,013	0,010	0,011	0,013	0,011	0,010		
	5	V	0,019	0,016	0,017	0,011	0,010	0,011	0,019	0,015	0,018	0,016	
		L	0,016	0,017	0,014	0,016	0,017	0,018	0,017	0,019	0,015		
	6	V	0,010	0,012	0,013	0,010	0,009	0,011	0,018	0,015	0,013	0,013	
		L	0,014	0,012	0,016	0,014	0,017	0,016	0,008	0,007	0,011		
	7	V	0,018	0,016	0,015	0,015	0,016	0,012	0,016	0,011	0,015	0,014	
		L	0,011	0,010	0,011	0,011	0,011	0,011	0,019	0,015	0,015		
	8	V	0,011	0,009	0,011	0,012	0,008	0,012	0,013	0,012	0,014	0,018	
		L	0,010	0,012	0,011	0,055	0,056	0,053	0,011	0,008	0,010		
	9	V	0,021	0,019	0,020	0,011	0,009	0,010	0,018	0,019	0,016	0,015	
		L	0,010	0,009	0,010	0,012	0,015	0,016	0,018	0,020	0,017		
	10	V	0,020	0,019	0,021	0,016	0,013	0,014	0,015	0,015	0,014	0,016	
		L	0,013	0,012	0,013	0,022	0,020	0,019	0,014	0,010	0,012		

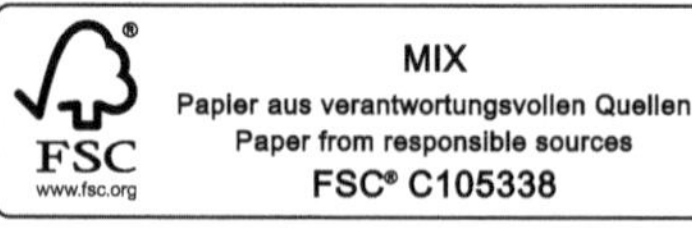

Printed by Books on Demand GmbH, Norderstedt / Germany